DIABETIC DIET AFTER 50 FOR BEGINNERS

Easy Low-Sugar Recipes for Optimal Wellbeing

By

Hector Wiggins

Table of Content

CHAPTER ONE

INTRODUCTION

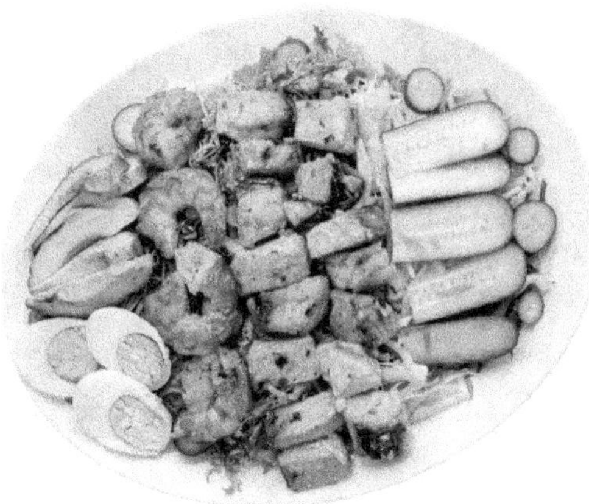

Welcome! If you've picked up this book, it's likely that you've recently been diagnosed with diabetes, or perhaps someone you care about has. The news can be overwhelming, especially if you're over 50 and find yourself navigating this new territory. You might be feeling a mix of emotions—confusion, worry, maybe even a bit of fear about what lies ahead. You're not alone, and we're here to help you through it.

This book is designed to be your trusted companion on this journey. We know that managing diabetes can seem daunting, but it doesn't have to be. Our goal is to provide you with clear, simple guidance on how to make lifestyle changes, particularly when it comes to diet, that will help you take control of your health. We believe that everyone deserves to live a dynamic and fulfilling life, and we want to help you achieve that by making informed choices that support your well-being.

We understand that changing habits isn't easy, especially when you're dealing with other aspects of life that come with age. But the good news is that by taking small, manageable steps, you can make a big difference in your health. In these pages, you'll find practical advice, delicious recipes, and tips on staying active that are designed specifically for people over 50. Whether you're just starting or looking to refine your approach, we've got you covered.

As you read through this book, you'll discover that a diabetic diet doesn't mean you have to give up all the foods you love. It's about finding a balance and making choices that work for you. By embracing these changes, you'll not only manage your diabetes more effectively but also enjoy a healthier and happier life.

Now that you've taken a deep breath, let's start this trip together. We're here to help you every step of the way, and you're at the perfect spot. Together, let's start down the path to a more promising and healthful future.

Understanding Diabetes

When you have diabetes, your body has problems controlling the amount of sugar, or glucose, in your blood. Normally, your body uses a hormone called insulin to help move sugar from your bloodstream into your cells, where it can be used for energy. In diabetes, this process doesn't work properly, leading to high levels of sugar in your blood.

Think of insulin as a key that unlocks the door to your cells, allowing sugar to enter. If the key doesn't work or is missing, the sugar stays in your bloodstream, leading to diabetes.

Types of Diabetes

There are three main types of diabetes: Type 1, Type 2, and gestational diabetes.

- **Type 1 Diabetes**: This type occurs when the body's immune system mistakenly attacks the cells in the pancreas that produce insulin. As a result, the body doesn't make insulin. This type usually appears in childhood or early adulthood and requires insulin injections to manage.

- **Type 2 Diabetes**: This type is more common and often develops in adults, although it's becoming more frequent in younger people. In Type 2 diabetes, the body either doesn't produce enough insulin or the cells don't respond to it properly (called insulin resistance). Lifestyle changes and medications can often help manage it.
- **Gestational Diabetes**: This type occurs during pregnancy and usually goes away after the baby is born. It may, however, raise the chance of Type 2 diabetes later in life.

Causes of Diabetes

The exact cause of diabetes depends on the type:

- Type 1 Diabetes is believed to be caused by an autoimmune response, where the body's immune system attacks insulin-producing cells. Genetics and environmental factors might play a role.
- Type 2 Diabetes is linked to lifestyle factors such as diet, physical activity, and obesity. Genetics also contribute, meaning it can run in families.

- Gestational Diabetes occurs due to hormonal changes during pregnancy that affect insulin's effectiveness.

Symptoms of Diabetes

Symptoms can vary depending on the type and how high blood sugar levels are. Common symptoms include:

1. Frequent urination
2. Excessive thirst
3. Increased hunger
4. Fatigue
5. Unexplained weight loss (more common in Type 1)
6. Blurred vision
7. Slow-healing sores or frequent infections
8. Hand or foot tingling or numbness (more common in Type 2).

Diagnosis of Diabetes

Diabetes is diagnosed through blood tests that measure your blood sugar levels:

- **Fasting Blood Glucose Test**: This measures your blood sugar after fasting for at least 8 hours.
- **Hemoglobin A1c Test**: This shows your average blood sugar levels over the past 2-3 months.
- **Oral Glucose Tolerance Test**: This checks your blood sugar before and after drinking a sugary solution.

Your doctor may use one or more of these tests to diagnose diabetes and determine its severity.

Treatment Options for Diabetes

Diabetes treatment varies according to type:
Type 1 Diabetes requires insulin therapy, which involves injecting insulin regularly. Insulin pumps and continuous glucose monitors are other options to help manage blood sugar.

Changes in lifestyle, including regular exercise, a nutritious diet, and weight loss, can effectively control type 2 diabetes. Prescriptions may also be written for medications, such as tablets or injectables. Insulin therapy may be required in certain circumstances.

Gestational Diabetes is managed with dietary changes and exercise. In some cases, insulin or other medications are required.

Managing Diabetes

Living with diabetes involves a combination of medical treatment, lifestyle changes, and self-care. Here are some key strategies:

- **Healthy Diet**: Focus on balanced meals with plenty of vegetables, whole grains, and lean proteins. Limit sugary foods and drinks. Work with a dietitian or diabetes educator for personalized advice.

- **Regular Exercise:** Aim for at least 150 minutes of moderate-intensity exercise per week, such as walking, swimming, or cycling. Exercise helps your body use insulin more effectively and keeps blood sugar levels stable.
- **Monitoring Blood Sugar**: If you have diabetes, you'll likely need to monitor your blood sugar regularly. This helps you understand how different foods, activities, and medications affect your blood sugar levels.
- **Medication and Insulin**: Follow your doctor's recommendations for medication and insulin use. If you're unsure about something, always ask your healthcare provider for clarification.
- **Routine Medical Check-ups**: Regular visits to your doctor help ensure your diabetes management plan is working and catch any complications early. You'll also need to monitor blood pressure, cholesterol, and other health indicators.

- **Stress Management:** Stress can affect blood sugar levels, so it's essential to find healthy ways to manage it. Try relaxation techniques, mindfulness, or hobbies that help you relax.

Common Myths and Misconceptions About Diabetes

Here are some common myths and misconceptions about diabetes:

Diabetes is caused by eating too much sugar. While diet plays a role, Type 1 diabetes is an autoimmune condition, and Type 2 diabetes involves a combination of factors, including genetics and lifestyle.
People with diabetes can't eat sweets. People with diabetes can enjoy sweets in moderation, but they need to be mindful of their overall diet and monitor blood sugar levels.
Diabetes is a death sentence.

People with diabetes can live long, healthy lives if their condition is properly managed. It's important to follow medical advice and make lifestyle changes to keep blood sugar levels in check.

Only overweight people get diabetes. While obesity is a risk factor for Type 2 diabetes, people of any weight can develop the condition. Type 1 diabetes is not related to body weight.

Reassuring Guidance for Those Newly Diagnosed or Living with Diabetes

If you've been diagnosed with diabetes or are living with the condition, remember that you're not alone. Many people successfully manage diabetes and live fulfilling lives. Here are some tips for navigating your diabetes journey:

- **Educate Yourself**: The more you know about diabetes, the better equipped you'll be to manage it. Read reputable sources, attend diabetes education classes, and ask your healthcare team questions.

- **Create a Support Network**: Assemble a team of family, friends, and medical experts who will stand with you. Consider joining a diabetes support group or connecting with others who have diabetes online.
- **Take One Step at a Time**: Managing diabetes can feel overwhelming at first, but you don't have to do everything at once. Start with small changes and gradually build healthier habits.
- **Prioritize Self-Care:** Taking care of yourself is crucial. Get enough sleep, eat well, exercise, and take time for relaxation. Self-care helps you stay balanced and better manage your diabetes.
- **Stay Positive**: Diabetes management can have ups and downs. Stay positive and remember that setbacks are part of the journey. Focus on progress, not perfection.

It is completely possible to manage diabetes with the correct strategy and assistance. Have self-compassion and ask for assistance when required.

Impact of Aging on Diabetes Management

The impact of aging on diabetes management involves a complex interplay of physiological, psychological, and social factors. As individuals age, they experience changes in their bodies, lifestyles, and health needs, all of which can influence how diabetes is managed. This comprehensive overview will cover the effects of aging on diabetes, the specific challenges faced by older adults, and the strategies to improve diabetes management in this population.

Physiological Changes with Aging

Aging brings about various physiological changes that can affect diabetes management:

- **Metabolic Changes**: As people age, their metabolism often slows down, which can impact glucose control and insulin sensitivity. This can lead to increased insulin resistance, making diabetes harder to manage.

- **Reduced Muscle Mass**: Sarcopenia, or age-related muscle loss, can affect glucose metabolism. Muscle tissue is a significant site for glucose uptake, so reduced muscle mass can contribute to increased blood sugar levels.
- **Changes in Body Composition**: Older adults often experience an increase in body fat, particularly visceral fat, which is associated with increased insulin resistance and cardiovascular risk.
- **Altered Organ Function**: Aging affects various organs involved in diabetes management, such as the kidneys and liver. This can impact medication metabolism and excretion, leading to altered drug effectiveness and an increased risk of side effects.

Challenges in Diabetes Management for Older Adults

Several challenges arise for older adults with diabetes:

- **Multiple Comorbidities**: Older adults often have multiple chronic conditions in addition to diabetes, such as hypertension, heart disease, and arthritis. Managing these comorbidities alongside diabetes can be complex and may require multiple medications, increasing the risk of drug interactions and adverse effects.
- **Cognitive Decline**: Aging is associated with a higher risk of cognitive impairment and dementia. Cognitive decline can affect an individual's ability to manage their diabetes, remember medication schedules, and follow dietary and exercise guidelines.
- **Functional Decline**: As individuals age, they may experience reduced mobility and functional abilities. This can impact their ability to exercise regularly, prepare healthy meals, and perform self-care tasks like blood glucose monitoring and insulin injections.

- **Sensory Impairments**: Age-related vision and hearing loss can complicate diabetes management. For example, vision problems can make it challenging to read medication labels or measure blood glucose levels accurately.
- **Social Isolation**: Older adults are at higher risk of social isolation and loneliness, which can impact mental health and make it more difficult to stay motivated with diabetes management routines.

Strategies for Effective Diabetes Management in Older Adults

To effectively manage diabetes in older adults, a multi-faceted approach is needed:
- **Personalized Care**: Diabetes management should be tailored to each individual's needs, taking into account their comorbidities, functional status, and cognitive abilities. A comprehensive geriatric assessment can help identify specific areas of concern.

- **Medication Management:** Careful consideration should be given to medication choices and dosages, with attention to potential drug interactions and side effects. Simplifying medication regimens can improve adherence.
- **Education and Support:** Providing diabetes education and support tailored to older adults can improve self-management skills. This may include support groups, caregiver involvement, and the use of technology to simplify diabetes care.
- **Diet and Nutrition:** Nutritional counseling should consider age-related changes in taste and appetite, as well as the need for a balanced diet that supports diabetes management and overall health. Meal planning assistance may be beneficial.
- **Exercise and Physical Activity:** Encouraging regular physical activity, within the individual's capabilities, can help manage blood glucose levels and improve overall health. Low-impact exercises like walking, swimming, or yoga may be suitable for older adults.

- **Addressing Social and Mental Health Needs:** Efforts to reduce social isolation and support mental health can improve diabetes management outcomes. This might include community programs, family involvement, and access to mental health resources.

Managing diabetes in older adults requires a comprehensive and adaptable approach. Understanding the physiological and functional changes that occur with aging, as well as the unique challenges faced by this population, is crucial. By adopting personalized strategies that consider these factors, healthcare providers and caregivers can support older adults in achieving better diabetes management and quality of life.

Setting Goals and Creating a Healthy Plan

As individuals reach the age of 50 and beyond, managing diabetes becomes increasingly important for maintaining overall health and well-being. A well-designed diabetic diet plan can play a crucial role in managing blood sugar levels, preventing complications, and promoting overall health. In this comprehensive guide, we'll explore setting goals and creating a healthy plan for a diabetic diet after 50.

Setting Goals:

- **Consultation with Healthcare Provider:** Begin by consulting with a healthcare provider or a registered dietitian who specializes in diabetes management. They can provide personalized advice based on individual health status, medications, and lifestyle factors.

- **Blood Sugar Targets**: Set specific, measurable blood sugar targets in consultation with healthcare professionals. These targets will guide dietary choices and overall management of diabetes.

- **Weight Management:** For individuals who are overweight or obese, setting realistic weight loss goals can significantly improve diabetes management. With a combination of food adjustments and increased exercise, aim for moderate weight loss.

- **Nutritional Goals**: Establish nutritional goals focusing on balanced meals that include a variety of nutrient-rich foods such as fruits, vegetables, whole grains, lean proteins, and healthy fats. Reduce your consumption of refined carbohydrates, processed foods, and saturated fats.

- **Physical Activity**: Incorporate regular physical activity into daily routines. Set achievable exercise goals based on individual fitness levels and preferences. Aim for a combination of aerobic exercises, strength training, and flexibility exercises to improve blood sugar control and overall health.

Creating a Healthy Diabetic Diet Plan:

- **Carbohydrate Management**: Focus on carbohydrate counting to regulate blood sugar levels. Select carbohydrates that are rich in fiber and have a gradual impact on blood sugar, such as whole, unprocessed foods, to maintain stable energy levels. Portion control is essential to avoid overconsumption of carbohydrates.

- **Balanced Meals**: Plan meals that include a balance of carbohydrates, proteins, and fats. Aim for consistent meal times and portion sizes to help stabilize blood sugar levels throughout the day.

- **Fiber-Rich Foods**: Include plenty of fiber-rich foods such as fruits, vegetables, legumes, and whole grains in the diet. Fiber helps regulate blood sugar levels, improves digestion, and promotes satiety.

- **Healthy Fats**: Incorporate sources of healthy fats such as avocados, nuts, seeds, and olive oil into the diet. These fats can lower the risk of heart disease and assist in increasing insulin sensitivity.

- **Limit Sodium and Processed Foods**: Reduce the intake of sodium and processed foods, which can contribute to hypertension and other complications associated with diabetes.

- **Hydration**: Drink water regularly throughout the day to stay hydrated. Cut back on sugary drinks and options for water, herbal teas, or flavorful infused water as healthier alternatives.

- **Meal Planning and Preparation**: Plan meals ahead of time and prepare healthy snacks to avoid impulsive food choices. Try different cooking techniques and dishes to make meals engaging and fun.

- **Monitor Blood Sugar Levels**: Regularly monitor blood sugar levels to track progress and make necessary adjustments to the meal plan. Keep a food diary to identify patterns and make informed decisions about dietary choices.

CHAPTER TWO

Basics of Diabetes Nutrition

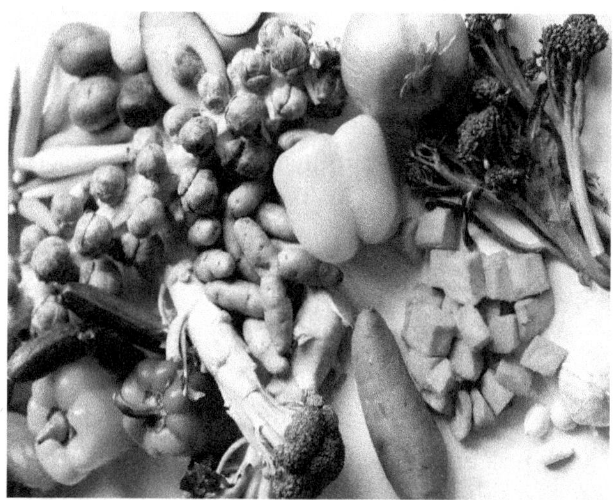

Maintaining a balanced diet is crucial for managing diabetes, especially as we age. If you are over 50 and diagnosed with diabetes, understanding the basics of diabetes nutrition can help you maintain your health and energy levels. Here's what you need to know to start building a diabetes-friendly diet.

1. **Understand Your Carbohydrates**

Carbohydrates have the most significant impact on blood sugar levels. As you age, it's essential to monitor carbohydrate intake and focus on complex carbohydrates over simple sugars. Aim for whole grains like brown rice, quinoa, and whole-wheat bread. Limit or avoid refined carbohydrates like white bread, pastries, and sugary drinks.

2. **Balance Your Plate**

The "plate method" is a simple guideline for creating balanced meals. Divide your plate into three sections: fill half with non-starchy vegetables (like leafy greens, broccoli, or bell peppers), one-quarter with lean proteins (like chicken, fish, or beans), and one-quarter with whole grains or starchy vegetables (like sweet potatoes). This method helps manage portion sizes and provides a variety of nutrients.

3. **Include Healthy Fats**

Fats can be part of a healthy diet, but it's important to choose the right kinds. Incorporate sources of unsaturated fats, like avocados, nuts, seeds, and olive oil, while limiting saturated and trans fats found in processed foods and fatty meats. These healthy fats can help improve heart health, which is particularly important for people with diabetes.

4. **Don't Forget Fiber**

Fiber is a valuable ally in the management of diabetes. It increases feelings of fullness and aids in blood sugar regulation. Make an effort to consume a diet rich in whole grains, legumes, fruits, and vegetables as well as other high-fiber foods. To prevent an upset stomach, gradually increase your intake of fiber while drinking lots of water.

5. **Monitor Your Portions**

Since metabolism slows down with age, portion control is essential to managing diabetes, especially in individuals over 50. To help you manage portion sizes, use smaller bowls and plates, and pay attention to the serving sizes on packaged items. Steer clear of eating directly out of big containers as this can result in overindulging.

6. **Limit Added Sugars and Processed Foods**

Cutting back on processed meals and added sugars is essential for diabetic care. These foods can contribute to weight gain by causing abrupt rises in blood sugar levels. When feasible, choose complete, unprocessed foods; if you do need a little sweetness, use stevia or monk fruit, which are natural sweeteners.

7. **Stay Hydrated**

Drinking enough water is crucial for good health and can assist in controlling blood sugar levels. Try to stay hydrated during the day by drinking lots of water and avoiding sugar-filled drinks like fruit juice and soda. Fruit or herb infusions added to water or herbal teas can enhance flavor without adding added sugar.

8. **Work with a Healthcare Professional**

Each person has unique nutritional demands, particularly when it comes to controlling a medical condition like diabetes. To create a customized nutrition plan, collaborate with a registered dietitian or certified diabetes educator. They can aid in goal-setting, progress monitoring, and diet modification as necessary.

After fifty, you may take charge of your health and enjoy a balanced diet by adhering to these fundamentals of diabetes nutrition. Recall that minor adjustments can have a big impact on your overall health and diabetes control.

Carbohydrates, Proteins, and Fats: What You Need to Know

Eating well is key to managing diabetes, especially as you age. If you're over 50 and diagnosed with diabetes, it's crucial to understand how carbohydrates, proteins, and fats affect your blood sugar levels and overall health. Here's a guide to help you navigate these macronutrients while keeping your diabetes in check.

Carbohydrates: The Main Focus for Blood Sugar Control Carbohydrates have the most direct impact on blood sugar, so they require careful management. But not every carbohydrate is made equal.

- **Complex Carbohydrates**: These carbs are absorbed more slowly and have a gentler effect on blood sugar. Good sources include whole grains (like quinoa, brown rice, and whole-wheat bread), legumes (like lentils and chickpeas), and starchy vegetables (like sweet potatoes and squash). Additionally, the high fiber content of these foods may aid in blood sugar regulation.

- **Simple Carbohydrates:** These carbs are quickly absorbed and can cause rapid spikes in blood sugar. They include refined grains, sugary snacks, candies, and soft drinks. It's best to limit or avoid these foods to maintain stable blood sugar levels.

Tip: Keep track of your carbohydrate intake by reading labels and using portion control. Many healthcare professionals recommend counting carbohydrates to help manage diabetes. A typical goal is to keep carbohydrate intake consistent throughout meals and snacks to avoid sudden fluctuations in blood sugar.

Proteins: Building Blocks for a Balanced Diet
Protein is vital for muscle maintenance, tissue repair, and satiety. Including adequate protein in your diet can help control blood sugar and support a healthy weight.

- **Lean Proteins**: Choose lean sources of protein such as chicken, fish, turkey, and low-fat dairy. Plant-based proteins like beans, lentils, and tofu are also excellent options, providing both protein and fiber.

- **Red Meat and Processed Meats**: These foods are high in saturated fat and cholesterol, which can increase the risk of heart disease—a common concern for people with diabetes. Limit red meat and avoid processed meats like bacon, sausage, and hot dogs.

Tip: Aim to include a source of protein in every meal and snack. It can help balance blood sugar levels and reduce hunger between meals.

Fats: Finding the Right Balance While fats are high in calories, they are essential for a healthy diet and can help improve blood sugar control when chosen wisely.

- **Healthy Fats**: Unsaturated fats from sources like avocados, nuts, seeds, and olive oil can benefit heart health. Omega-3 fatty acids, found in fatty fish like salmon and mackerel, can also reduce inflammation and lower the risk of cardiovascular disease.

- **Unhealthy Fats**: Saturated and trans fats, found in fried foods, processed snacks, and fatty cuts of meat, can increase bad cholesterol levels and the risk of heart disease. Limit these fats to maintain heart health.

Tip: Incorporate healthy fats into your meals but be mindful of portion sizes, as fats are calorie-dense. Use cooking methods that don't require excess fat, like baking, grilling, or steaming.

Additional Considerations Portion Control: Controlling portion sizes is essential for both blood sugar regulation and weight loss. Downsize your tableware - use smaller plates, bowls, and utensils to help control portion sizes and develop healthy eating habits.

Hydration: Stay hydrated with water, unsweetened beverages, and herbal teas. Steer clear of sugary beverages that could elevate blood sugar.

Meal Planning and Preparation: Planning meals and snacks in advance can help you make healthier choices and maintain consistency in your diet.

Glycemic Index and Glycemic Load

Understanding Glycemic Index (GI)
The Glycemic Index (GI) gauges how quickly blood
sugar levels are raised by carbs in food in relation to
pure glucose, which has a GI of 100. Foods with a
high GI are rapidly digested and absorbed, causing
spikes in blood sugar levels.

Understanding Glycemic Load (GL)
The term Glycemic Load (GL) describes how much
and what kind of carbs are included in a meal. It's
calculated by multiplying the GI of a food by the
amount of carbohydrates in a serving and dividing
by 100. GL gives a more accurate picture of how a
food affects blood sugar levels than GI alone.

GI vs GL: What's the Difference?
While GI measures how quickly a
carbohydrate-containing food raises blood sugar,
GL considers both the quality and quantity of
carbohydrates consumed. Therefore, GL provides a
more comprehensive understanding of how a food
affects blood sugar levels.

How to Use GI and GL for Blood Sugar Management

For better blood sugar management, aim to consume foods with a low to moderate GI and GL. These foods are digested and absorbed more slowly, leading to gradual increases in blood sugar levels. Pairing carbohydrates with protein, fiber, and healthy fats can also help slow down digestion and reduce the overall glycemic impact of a meal.

The Impact of GI and GL on Weight and Health

High-GI and GL diets have been associated with an increased risk of obesity, type 2 diabetes, and heart disease. Foods with a lower GI and GL tend to be higher in fiber and nutrients, which can help with weight management and overall health.

GI and GL Values of Common Foods

Here are some examples of common foods and their GI and GL values:

Low GI and GL foods: Non-starchy vegetables, legumes, whole grains (e.g., barley, quinoa), fruits (e.g., berries, apples), nuts, and seeds.

Moderate GI and GL foods: Whole grain bread, brown rice, oatmeal, sweet potatoes, and some fruits (e.g., bananas, grapes).
High GI and GL foods: White bread, white rice, sugary cereals, soda, candy, and processed snacks.

Incorporating GI and GL into Your Meal Plan
When planning meals, focus on incorporating a variety of low to moderate GI and GL foods. Ample amounts of nutritious grains, lean meats, healthy fats, and non-starchy veggies should be included. Pay attention to portion sizes and consider pairing high-GI foods with lower-GI options to balance out the meal.

Common Myths and Misconceptions About GI and GL

- **Myth**: All carbohydrates are bad for blood sugar control.
- **Fact**: Not all carbohydrates are created equal. Choosing whole, minimally processed carbohydrates with a low to moderate GI and GL can support better blood sugar management and overall health.

- **Myth**: You should completely avoid high-GI foods.
- **Fact**: While it's beneficial to limit high-GI foods, they can still be enjoyed in moderation, especially when paired with lower-GI foods to minimize their glycemic impact.

In summary, understanding and incorporating GI and GL into your diet can be a valuable tool for managing blood sugar levels, promoting weight management, and improving overall health, especially for individuals over 50 with diabetes. By making informed food choices and balancing your meals with a variety of nutrient-rich foods, you can support your health and well-being for years to come.

Portion Control and Meal Planning

Diabetes can bring distinct difficulties, particularly as we get older. However, controlling diabetes may be empowering and enhance general health and well-being if the appropriate information and techniques are applied. This thorough book will provide personalized recommendations and useful pointers for people over 50 who have diabetes, with an emphasis on meal planning and portion management. Together, let's set out on a journey to better diabetes care, encompassing everything from recognizing dietary requirements to controlling blood sugar levels and overcoming typical obstacles.

Recognizing Your Specific Nutritional Needs:
Our bodies change as we age, resulting in changes to our metabolism and dietary needs. It's critical to identify these changes in older persons with diabetes and modify dietary choices accordingly. Important things to think about are:

- **Protein:** Aim for lean protein sources such as poultry, fish, tofu, and legumes to support muscle health and blood sugar control.
- **Fiber**: Incorporate fiber-rich foods like vegetables, fruits, whole grains, and legumes to promote digestive health and regulate blood sugar levels.
- **Healthy Fats**: Choose sources of healthy fats such as avocados, nuts, seeds, and olive oil to support heart health and provide sustained energy.

Managing Blood Sugar Levels through Portion Control and Meal Planning:

Portion control plays a vital role in managing blood sugar levels effectively. By keeping portions in check and balancing macronutrients, you can prevent spikes and dips in blood glucose.

Here are some practical tips:

- **Plate Method**: Visualize your plate divided into sections: half filled with non-starchy vegetables, a quarter with lean protein, and a quarter with whole grains or starchy vegetables.

- **Use Smaller Plates**: Option for smaller
  plates to naturally control portion sizes and
  avoid overeating.
- **Read Food Labels**: Pay attention to serving
  sizes and carbohydrate content on food
  labels to make informed choices.

Creating a Personalized Eating Plan:
No two individuals are the same, and a
one-size-fits-all approach to meal planning may not
be effective. Work with a healthcare provider or
registered dietitian to develop a personalized eating
plan that considers factors such as medication
schedules, physical activity levels, and health goals.
Your eating plan should be flexible, realistic, and
sustainable for long-term success.

Healthy Eating Habits and Food Choices:
Incorporate these healthy eating habits and food
choices into your daily routine:

- **Hydration:** Stay hydrated by drinking
  plenty of water throughout the day, and limit
  sugary beverages.

Eating Slowly, Savoring Every Bite, and Observing Fullness and Hunger Cues are all examples of Mindful Eating.

- **Snack Smart**: Choose nutritious snacks such as fresh fruit, yogurt, nuts, or vegetables with hummus to keep blood sugar levels stable between meals.

Managing Carbohydrate Intake and Counting Carbs:

Counting carbohydrates is a useful technique for controlling blood sugar levels. Keep these tips in mind:

- **Choose Complex Carbs**: Option for whole grains, fruits, and vegetables over refined carbohydrates to provide sustained energy and fiber.
- **Monitor Portions**: Be mindful of portion sizes when consuming carbohydrate-rich foods, and spread them evenly throughout the day to prevent blood sugar spikes.

Dealing with Common Challenges:
Living with diabetes may present various challenges, but with the right strategies, you can overcome them:

- **Medication Side Effects**: Discuss any medication side effects with your healthcare provider, and explore alternative options if necessary.
- **Digestive Issues**: Choose easily digestible foods and consider smaller, more frequent meals if you experience digestive issues such as bloating or discomfort.
- **Social Eating Pressures**: Communicate your dietary needs with friends and family, and suggest healthier alternatives when dining out or attending social gatherings.

Sample Meal Plans and Recipes:

Here are sample meal plans and recipes tailored to older adults with diabetes:

- **Breakfast:** Greek yogurt with berries and almonds, whole grain toast with avocado.
- **Lunch**: Grilled chicken salad with mixed greens, vegetables, and vinaigrette dressing.
- Dinner is baked salmon paired with roasted veggies and quinoa.

Advice on Cooking, Grocery Shopping, and Dining Out:

Navigate grocery shopping, cooking, and eating out with these tips:

- **Make a List:** Plan your meals and make a list before heading to the grocery store to avoid impulse purchases.
- **Cook in Batches**: Prepare meals in advance and freeze individual portions for quick and convenient meals.

- **Eating Out**: Look for restaurants that offer healthier options, and don't hesitate to customize your order to meet your dietary needs.

In summary, managing diabetes through portion control and meal planning is a journey that requires patience, dedication, and support. By understanding your unique nutritional needs, adopting healthy eating habits, and seeking guidance from healthcare professionals, you can take control of your health and thrive with diabetes. Remember, you're not alone on this journey, and every small step towards better diabetes management counts.

CHAPTER THREE

Creating a Diabetes Diet After 50

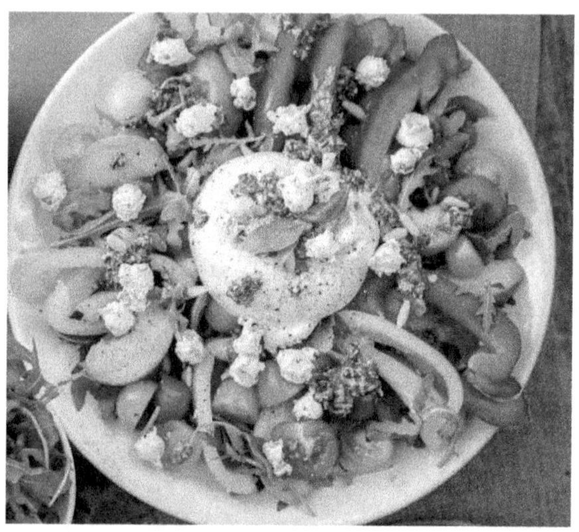

Managing diabetes after 50 calls for a customized dietary plan. With the practical advice in this guide, you can create a diet plan that works for you and enable you to effectively manage your illness and lead a fulfilling life.

Taking Control of Your Diet After 50:

- Emphasize the importance of proactive management through diet.
- Highlight the role of diet in controlling blood sugar levels and preventing complications.
- Encourage a positive mindset towards making sustainable dietary changes.

Setting Realistic Goals and Seeking Professional Guidance:
- Stress the significance of setting achievable objectives in managing diabetes.
- Advocate for consulting healthcare providers or registered dietitians to develop personalized strategies.
- Discuss the benefits of ongoing support and monitoring.

Assessing Your Current Eating Habits:
- Encourage self-reflection on current dietary patterns and habits.
- Provide guidance on keeping a food diary to track intake and identify areas for improvement.

- Address common pitfalls such as excessive sugar consumption and irregular meal times.

Creating a Balanced Meal Plan:
- Explain the importance of balancing macronutrients, including carbohydrates, protein, and fats.
- Discuss the concepts of glycemic index and glycemic load in food selection.
- Highlight the role of fiber and water intake in managing blood sugar levels and promoting overall health.
- Emphasize the inclusion of healthy fats and omega-3s for heart health and inflammation control.
- Address potential vitamin and mineral deficiencies common in older adults with diabetes.

Including Foods That Are Good for Diabetes:

- Provide a list of nutrient-rich foods suitable for diabetes management, such as leafy greens, berries, nuts, and fatty fish.
- Discuss the benefits of whole grains and legumes in stabilizing blood sugar levels and promoting satiety.

Managing Carbohydrate Intake:
- Explain the importance of carbohydrate counting in diabetes management.
- Provide practical tips for estimating portion sizes and reading food labels.
- Discuss strategies for incorporating carbohydrates into meals while controlling blood sugar levels.

Overcoming Common Challenges:
- Address potential medication side effects and their impact on appetite and digestion.
- Provide solutions for managing digestive issues commonly associated with diabetes.
- Offer strategies for navigating social situations and dining out while adhering to dietary restrictions.

Sample Meal Plans and Recipes:
- Provide a range of sample meal plans that are adapted to the dietary requirements of elderly diabetics.
- Include easy-to-make, tasty recipes with ingredients that are safe for diabetics.

In summary, Understanding your own health demands and lifestyle is the first step towards taking control of your diabetes diet after 50. You can successfully manage your disease and have a full, active life by establishing realistic goals, getting professional advice, and making educated dietary decisions. Recall that creating a customized eating plan that suits you requires speaking with medical professionals or trained dietitians.

Importance of Regular Monitoring and Blood Sugar Management

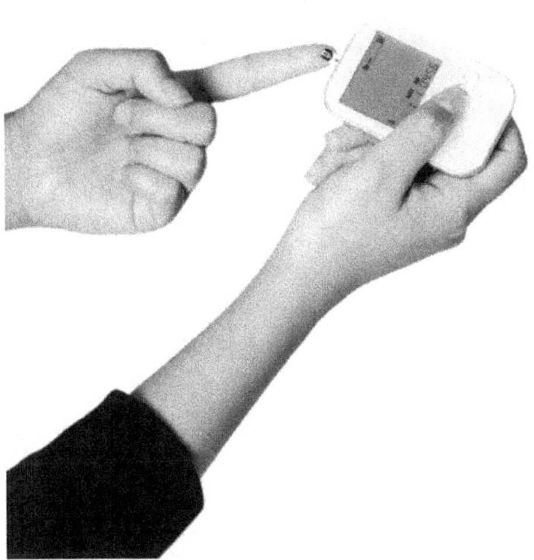

Managing diabetes after 50 requires a comprehensive approach, with regular monitoring of blood sugar levels playing a crucial role in maintaining health and preventing complications. This article explores the importance of consistent monitoring and effective blood sugar management in the context of a diabetic diet tailored for individuals over 50.

Understanding the Significance of Regular Monitoring:
- Highlight the dynamic nature of blood sugar levels and their impact on overall health.
- Emphasize the importance of frequent monitoring to track changes and adjust dietary and lifestyle strategies accordingly.
- Discuss the role of self-monitoring in empowering individuals to take control of their health.

Maintaining Stable Blood Sugar Levels:
- Explain the implications of fluctuating blood sugar levels, including short-term symptoms and long-term complications.
- Advocate for proactive management through dietary choices, physical activity, and medication adherence.
- Stress the importance of personalized blood sugar targets and individualized management plans.

Strategies for Effective Blood Sugar Management:

- Discuss the principles of glycemic control, including carbohydrate counting, portion control, and meal timing.
- Highlight the importance of balanced nutrition, with a focus on whole foods, fiber-rich carbohydrates, lean proteins, and healthy fats.
- Encourage regular physical activity as a means of improving insulin sensitivity and promoting blood sugar regulation.
- Address the role of medication, insulin therapy, or other treatment modalities in achieving optimal blood sugar control.

Importance of Timely Intervention and Adjustment:

- Emphasize the need for proactive intervention in response to changes in blood sugar levels, medication regimens, or lifestyle factors.
- Discuss the value of regular follow-up appointments with healthcare providers or diabetes educators to review progress and make necessary adjustments.

- Provide guidance on recognizing signs of hyperglycemia or hypoglycemia and implementing appropriate interventions.

Monitoring Beyond Blood Sugar Levels:
- Highlight the importance of comprehensive health monitoring, including blood pressure, cholesterol levels, and kidney function, in individuals with diabetes.
- Discuss the interconnectedness of various health parameters and their collective impact on overall well-being.

In summary, regular monitoring of blood sugar levels and diligent management are cornerstone principles in the diabetic diet after 50. By staying vigilant, making informed choices, and seeking support from healthcare professionals, individuals can optimize their health outcomes and enjoy a fulfilling life despite the challenges posed by diabetes. Remember, consistency and proactive management are key to long-term success in diabetes care.

Adjusting Dietary Intake to Age-Related Changes

Beyond the age of fifty, people's bodies experience a variety of changes that may have an impact on their nutritional requirements, especially for those who are treating diabetes. Maintaining good health and controlling blood sugar levels require an understanding of these changes and the ability to adjust to them. The following are some tips for modifying your food intake to account for age-related changes:

Increased Protein Intake for Muscle Health: Aging is often accompanied by a decline in muscle mass, known as sarcopenia. To combat this, older adults should aim to increase their protein intake. Include sources of lean protein such as poultry, fish, tofu, beans, and lentils in your meals. For general health, muscle upkeep, and repair, protein is necessary.

Choosing Complex Carbohydrates for Sustained Energy: Aging can affect the body's ability to process carbohydrates and regulate blood sugar levels. Option for complex carbohydrates like whole grains, fruits, vegetables, and legumes, which provide fiber and slow-release energy. These foods can help maintain blood sugar levels and provide you steady energy all day long.

Including Good Fats for Heart and Brain Health: Changes in lipid metabolism and a higher risk of cardiovascular disease are linked to aging. Add foods like avocados, almonds, seeds, and olive oil to your diet as sources of good fats. These fats promote heart health, mental clarity, and general well-being.

Staying Hydrated and Managing Fluid Intake: Aging can affect the body's ability to regulate fluid balance and thirst sensation. It's essential for older adults to stay hydrated by drinking plenty of water throughout the day. Limit sugary beverages and caffeinated drinks, which can have diuretic effects and contribute to dehydration.

Considering Supplements and Vitamins:
As we age, nutrient absorption may decline, and certain vitamins and minerals may become deficient. Consult with your healthcare provider or a registered dietitian about supplementing with nutrients like vitamin D and calcium, which are crucial for bone health. Additionally, older adults with diabetes may benefit from supplements such as magnesium and B vitamins to support blood sugar regulation.

After the age of fifty, you can continue to improve general health, effectively control diabetes, and maintain optimal well-being by modifying your dietary consumption to account for age-related changes. Never forget to seek the advice of medical professionals for specific dietary guidelines and help when managing your diabetes.

Including Fiber and Whole Grains

Adding fiber-rich foods and whole grains into your diabetic diet after the age of 50 is important for managing blood sugar levels, supporting digestive health, and reducing the risk of long-term conditions such as heart disease and stroke. Here's why fiber and whole grains are beneficial and how to include them in your meals:

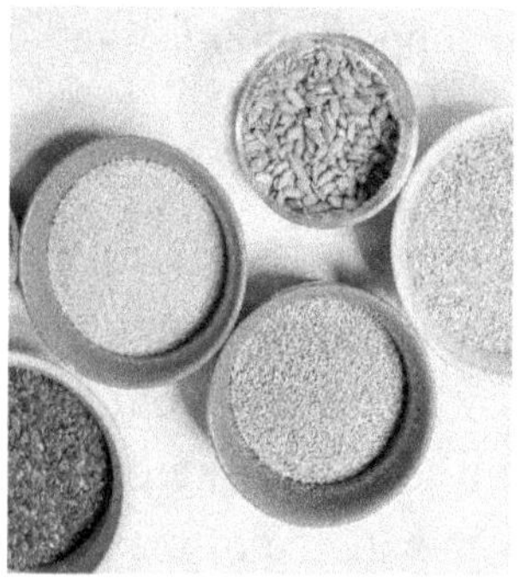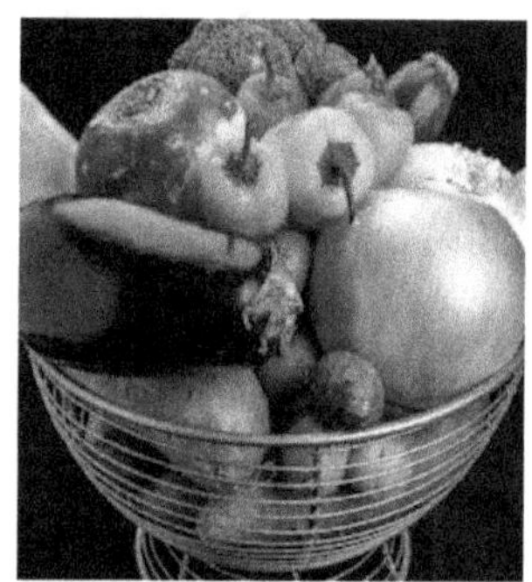

Benefits of Fiber:

- **Blood Sugar Control**: Fiber reduces the rate at which glucose is absorbed, which helps to avoid sharp rises in blood sugar following meals. This is particularly important for individuals with diabetes in maintaining stable blood sugar levels throughout the day.

- **Weight Management**: High-fiber foods are often lower in calories and can help you feel full and satisfied for longer periods, reducing the likelihood of overeating and promoting weight loss or weight management.

- **Heart Health**: Soluble fiber found in foods like oats, beans, and fruits can help lower cholesterol levels, reducing the risk of heart disease and stroke.

Benefits of Whole Grains:
- **Stable Blood Sugar Levels:** Whole grains contain complex carbohydrates, which are digested more slowly than refined grains. This gradual digestion helps prevent rapid spikes and crashes in blood sugar levels, making them an excellent choice for individuals with diabetes.
- **Rich in Nutrients:** Whole grains are a good source of essential nutrients such as fiber, vitamins, minerals, and antioxidants, which are vital for overall health and well-being.

- **Digestive Health**: The fiber content in whole grains promotes regular bowel movements, prevents constipation, and supports a healthy digestive system.

How to Include Fiber and Whole Grains in Your Diet:

- Choose Whole Grain Options: Replace refined grains like white bread, pasta, and rice with whole grain alternatives such as whole wheat bread, brown rice, quinoa, barley, and oats. Look for products labeled "whole grain" or "100% whole wheat" to ensure you're getting the full nutritional benefits.
- **Start Your Day with Fiber:** Enjoy a fiber-rich breakfast by incorporating foods like whole grain cereal, oatmeal, or whole wheat toast with avocado or nut butter. Add fruits such as berries or bananas for an extra boost of fiber and flavor.

- **Snack Smart**: Option for whole grain snacks such as air-popped popcorn, whole grain crackers with hummus or cheese, or a piece of fruit with nuts or seeds. These snacks provide a satisfying crunch and a dose of fiber to keep you feeling full between meals.

- **Bulk Up Your Meals**: Add fiber-rich vegetables like broccoli, Brussels sprouts, spinach, and kale to your meals. These vegetables not only provide fiber but also add volume and nutrients without adding excess calories.

- **Experiment with Ancient Grains**: Explore ancient grains like quinoa, farro, amaranth, and bulgur to add variety to your diet. These grains offer unique flavors, textures, and nutritional profiles, making them a versatile and nutritious addition to meals.

Including fiber and whole grains in your diabetic diet after the age of 50 can contribute to better blood sugar control, improved digestive health, and overall well-being. Be sure to gradually increase your fiber intake and drink plenty of water to prevent digestive discomfort. Consult with a healthcare provider or registered dietitian for personalized recommendations and guidance on incorporating fiber and whole grains into your diet plan.

CHAPTER FOUR

Meal Planning And Recipes

Tips for Meal Planning and Grocery Shopping

Plan Ahead: Schedule time for meal planning and create a weekly menu to ensure balanced nutrition.

Choose Whole Foods: Option for fresh fruits, vegetables, lean proteins, and whole grains over processed foods.

Read Labels: Check food labels for added sugars, sodium, and unhealthy fats. Aim for low-sugar and low-sodium options.

Portion Control: Be mindful of portion sizes to manage blood sugar levels effectively.

Stock Up on Staples: Keep pantry essentials like canned beans, whole grains, nuts, and seeds for quick and healthy meals.

Breakfast Recipes

Oatmeal with Fruit and Nuts:

- **Ingredients**: Rolled oats, unsweetened almond milk, mixed berries, chopped nuts (almonds, walnuts), cinnamon.
- **Instructions**: Cook oats with almond milk, top with berries, nuts, and a sprinkle of cinnamon.

Greek Yogurt Parfait:

- **Ingredients**: Greek yogurt, mixed berries, chopped nuts, drizzle of honey or maple syrup (optional).
- **Instructions**: Layer yogurt, berries, and nuts in a glass. Drizzle with honey if desired.

Lunch Recipes

Grilled Chicken Salad with Avocado:

- **Ingredients**: Grilled chicken breast, mixed greens, cherry tomatoes, cucumber, avocado, balsamic vinaigrette.
- **Instructions:** Toss ingredients together and top with sliced avocado. Drizzle with balsamic vinaigrette.

Lentil Soup with Whole Grain Bread:

- **Ingredients**: Lentils, carrots, celery, onion, garlic, low-sodium vegetable broth, whole grain bread.
- **Instructions**: Sauté vegetables, add lentils and broth, simmer until tender. Serve with whole grain bread.

Dinner Recipes

Baked Salmon with Roasted Vegetables and Quinoa:

- **Ingredients**: Salmon filets, mixed vegetables (bell peppers, zucchini, broccoli), olive oil, lemon juice, quinoa.
- **Instructions:** Season salmon, roast with vegetables tossed in olive oil and lemon juice. Serve with cooked quinoa.

Vegetable Stir-Fry with Tofu and Brown Rice:

- **Ingredients:** Firm tofu, mixed vegetables (bell peppers, snap peas, carrots), low-sodium soy sauce, garlic, ginger, brown rice.
- **Instructions**: Stir-fry tofu and vegetables with garlic and ginger. Serve with soy sauce over brown rice.

Snack Ideas

- Carrot Sticks with Hummus
- Apple Slices with Almond Butter

Cooking Methods and Techniques for Older Adults

- **Slow Cooking:** Utilize slow cookers for easy, hands-off cooking.
- **One-Pot Meals**: Minimize cleanup by preparing meals that require only one pot or pan.
- **Prepare in Advance**: Chop vegetables and portion ingredients ahead of time for quicker meal preparation.
- **Easy Chewing Options**: Cook or steam vegetables until tender, and choose softer proteins like fish and tofu.

Ingredient Substitutions and Variations

- **Sweeteners**: Use natural sweeteners like stevia or monk fruit instead of refined sugars.
- **Grains**: Substitute white rice and pasta with whole grains like quinoa, brown rice, or whole wheat pasta.
- **Proteins**: Replace meat with plant-based proteins like beans, lentils, or tofu for meatless options.

Nutritional Information and Carb Counting Guidance

- **Portion Control**: Measure portions to manage carbohydrate intake and blood sugar levels.
- **Balanced Meals**: Aim for meals that contain a mix of carbohydrates, proteins, and healthy fats.
- **Consult a Dietitian**: Seek guidance from a registered dietitian for personalized carb counting and meal planning advice.

Sample Meal Plans and Grocery Lists

Sample Meal Plan:
- **Breakfast**: Greek Yogurt Parfait
- **Lunch**: Lentil Soup with Whole Grain Bread
- **Dinner**: Baked Salmon with Roasted Vegetables and Quinoa
- **Snacks:** Apple slices with almond butter and carrot sticks with hummus.

Grocery List:
- Rolled oats
- Unsweetened almond milk
- Mixed berries
- Chopped nuts (almonds, walnuts)
- Cinnamon
- Greek yogurt
- Avocado
- Grilled chicken breast
- Mixed greens
- Cherry tomatoes
- Cucumber

- Lentils

- Carrots
- Celery
- Onion
- Garlic
- Low-sodium vegetable broth
- Whole grain bread
- Salmon filets
- Mixed vegetables (bell peppers, zucchini, broccoli)
- Olive oil
- Lemon juice
- Quinoa
- Firm tofu
- Snap peas
- Low-sodium soy sauce
- Ginger

By following these guidelines and recipes, individuals with diabetes over 50 can enjoy delicious, easy-to-prepare meals that meet their nutritional needs and support their overall health and well-being.

Breakfast Recipes for Diabetics

Breakfast is the most important meal of the day, especially for individuals with diabetes. A nutritious breakfast sets the tone for stable blood sugar levels and provides essential nutrients to fuel the body for the day ahead. In this guide, we'll explore 10 breakfast recipes specifically designed for those managing diabetes. These recipes are low in added sugars and refined carbohydrates, high in fiber and protein, rich in healthy fats and nutrients, easy to prepare, and versatile to accommodate various dietary needs and preferences.

Omelet with Vegetables and Whole Grain Toast:

- **Ingredients**: Eggs, bell peppers, onions, spinach, whole grain bread.
- **Instructions**: Whisk eggs, add diced vegetables, cook in a non-stick pan. Serve with toasted whole grain bread.

- **Tips**: Customize with your favorite vegetables like mushrooms, tomatoes, or broccoli. Use egg whites for a lower-fat option.

Greek Yogurt with Berries and Nuts:

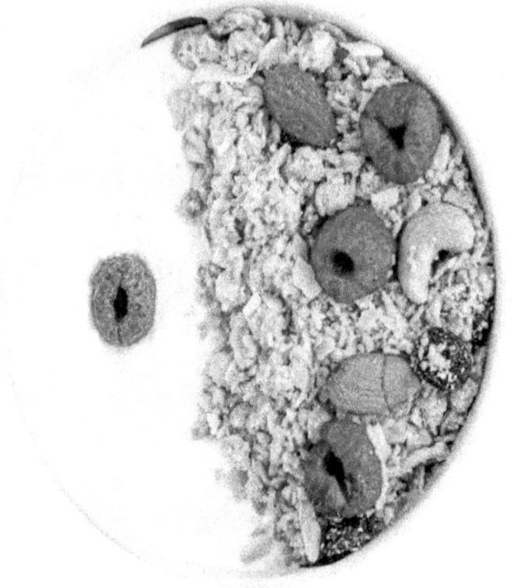

- **Ingredients**: Greek yogurt, mixed berries, almonds or walnuts.
- **Instructions**: Mix yogurt with berries and top with nuts.
- **Tips**: Choose plain Greek yogurt to avoid added sugars. Substitute nuts with seeds like chia or flax for variety.

Avocado Toast with Scrambled Eggs:

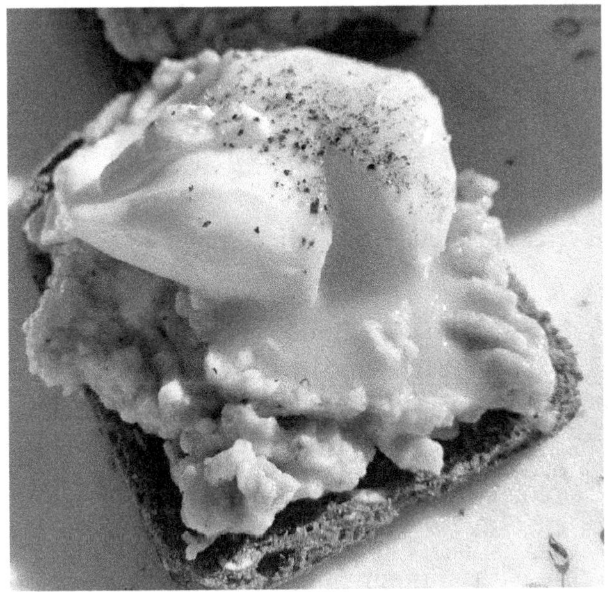

- **Ingredients**: Whole grain bread, avocado, eggs.
- **Instructions**: Mash avocado on toasted bread. Scramble eggs and serve on top.

- **Tips**: Add a sprinkle of chili flakes or black pepper for extra flavor. Swap bread with whole grain English muffins or rice cakes.

Whole Grain Toast served with a spinach and feta omelet:

- **Ingredients**: Eggs, spinach, feta cheese, whole grain bread.
- **Instructions**: Cook spinach in a pan until wilted. Whisk eggs, add spinach and crumbled feta, cook as an omelet. Serve with whole grain toast.
- **Tips**: Experiment with different cheeses like goat cheese or mozzarella. Add diced tomatoes or olives for extra flavor.

Smoothie with Spinach and Almond Milk:

- **Ingredients**: Spinach, banana, almond milk, protein powder (optional).
- **Instructions**: Blend spinach, banana, and almond milk until smooth. Add protein powder if desired.

- **Tips**: Incorporate other fruits like berries or mango for variety. Include a handful of nuts or seeds for added protein and healthy fats.

Black beans with scrambled eggs in a breakfast burrito:

- **Ingredients**: Whole grain tortilla, eggs, black beans, diced tomatoes, avocado.
- **Instructions**: Scramble eggs, heat black beans, and assemble burrito with desired toppings.
- **Tips**: Use low-carb or whole wheat tortillas for a healthier option. Add salsa or hot sauce for extra flavor without added sugars.

Fresh Fruit and Coconut Milk Chia Seed Pudding:

- **Ingredients**: Chia seeds, coconut milk, fresh fruit (e.g., berries, mango).
- **Instructions**: Stir chia seeds into coconut milk and let aside to chill. Serve topped with fresh fruit.

- **Tips**: Sweeten with a drizzle of honey or maple syrup if desired. Experiment with different types of milk like almond or oat milk.

Whole Grain Cereal with Almond Milk and Sliced Banana:

- **Ingredients**: Whole grain cereal, almond milk, banana.
- **Instructions**: Pour cereal into a bowl, add almond milk, top with sliced banana.
- **Tips**: Look for cereals with minimal added sugars and high fiber content. Substitute banana with other fruits like apples or berries.

Quinoa Breakfast Bowl with Roasted Vegetables and Poached Eggs:

- **Ingredients**: Quinoa, roasted vegetables (e.g., sweet potatoes, broccoli), poached eggs.

- **Instructions**: Cook quinoa, roast vegetables, poach eggs, and assemble in a bowl.
- **Tips**: Make extra quinoa and roasted vegetables for easy meal prep. Top with a drizzle of olive oil or balsamic glaze for added flavor.

Whole Grain Waffles Served with Yogurt and Fresh Fruit:

- **Ingredients**: Whole grain waffle mix, fresh fruit (e.g., strawberries, blueberries), Greek yogurt.
- **Instructions**: Prepare waffle batter, cook waffles, and serve with fresh fruit and a dollop of Greek yogurt.
- **Tips**: Add a sprinkle of cinnamon or nutmeg to the waffle batter for extra flavor. Use unsweetened Greek yogurt to avoid added sugars.

Meal Planning and Grocery Shopping Tips:

- Plan your breakfasts ahead of time to ensure you have all the necessary ingredients.

- Create a grocery list and follow it to prevent impulsive buys.
- Choose whole, unprocessed foods whenever possible.
- Option for fresh or frozen fruits and vegetables over canned varieties to minimize added sugars and sodium.

Substitutions and Variations:

- Change the ingredients according to your dietary needs and tastes.
- Experiment with different combinations of fruits, vegetables, proteins, and grains to keep breakfasts interesting.
- Use alternative sweeteners like stevia or monk fruit extract instead of sugar.

With these delicious and healthy breakfast recipes, individuals with diabetes can start their day on the right foot. By focusing on whole foods that are low in added sugars and refined carbohydrates, high in fiber and protein, and rich in healthy fats and nutrients, you can support stable blood sugar levels and overall well-being. Remember to personalize these recipes to suit your tastes and dietary needs, and enjoy the benefits of a nutritious breakfast every day.

Lunch and Snack Recipes for Diabetics

Lunch

Grilled Salmon with Asparagus and Quinoa

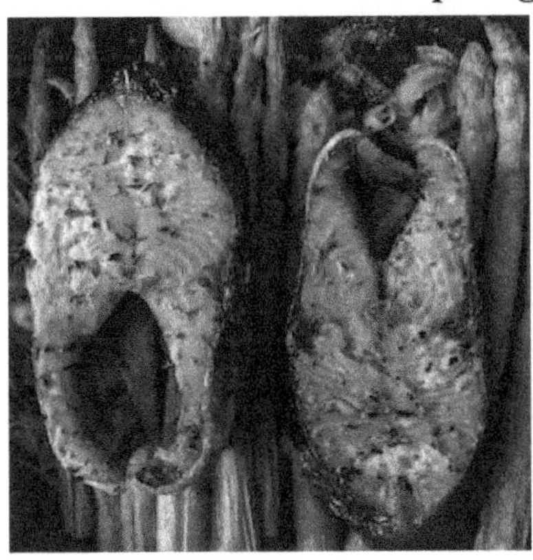

- **Ingredients**: Salmon filets, asparagus spears, quinoa, olive oil, lemon juice, garlic, salt, and pepper.
- **Instructions**: Marinate salmon in olive oil, lemon juice, garlic, salt, and pepper. Grill salmon and asparagus until cooked. Cook quinoa separately. Serve grilled salmon and asparagus over quinoa.

Turkey and Avocado Wrap

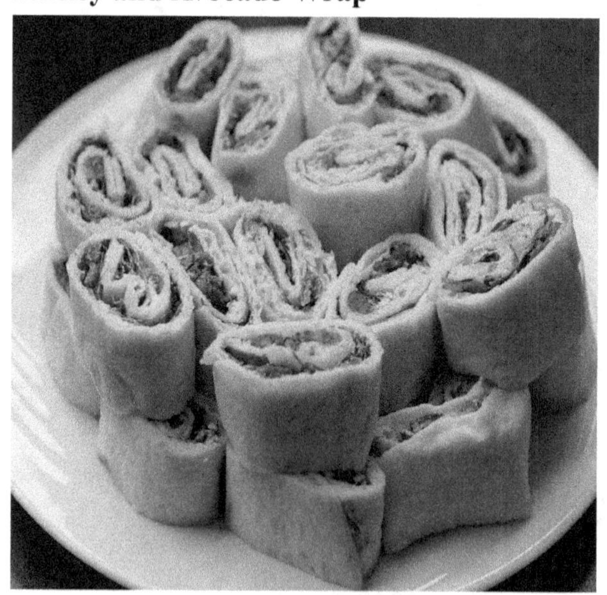

- **Ingredients**: Whole grain tortillas, sliced turkey breast, avocado, lettuce, tomato, and mustard.
- **Instructions:** Lay out tortillas, spread mustard, add turkey, avocado, lettuce, and tomato. Tightly roll, then cut in half.

Vegetable Stir-Fry with Tofu

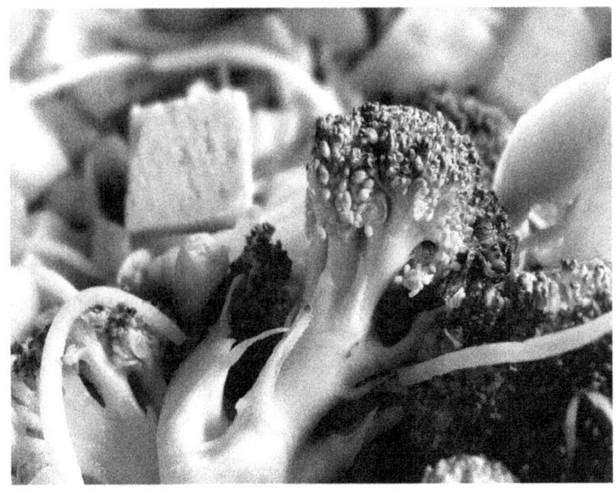

- **Ingredients**: Tofu, mixed vegetables (bell peppers, broccoli, carrots, snap peas),

low-sodium soy sauce, garlic, ginger, olive oil.
- **Instructions**: Press tofu to remove excess moisture. Stir-fry tofu and vegetables in olive oil with garlic and ginger. Vegetables should be cooked until softened by adding soy sauce.

Quinoa Salad with Chickpeas and Veggies

- **Ingredients**: Cooked quinoa, chickpeas, cherry tomatoes, cucumber, red onion, feta cheese, lemon juice, olive oil, salt, and pepper.
- **Instructions**: Mix all ingredients together in a bowl. Drizzle with lemon juice and olive oil. Season with salt and pepper.

Chicken and Vegetable Skewers

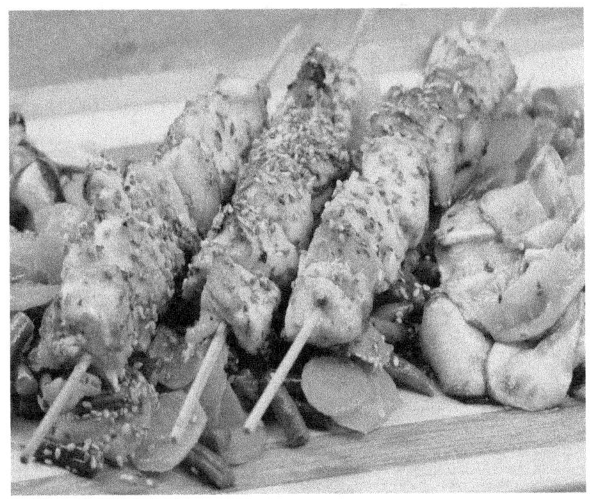

- **Ingredients**: Chicken breast, bell peppers, zucchini, cherry tomatoes, olive oil, lemon juice, garlic, salt, and pepper.
- **Instructions**: Cut chicken and vegetables into cubes. Marinate in olive oil, lemon juice, garlic, salt, and pepper. After putting onto skewers, cook under the grill.

Spinach and Feta Stuffed Chicken Breast

- **Ingredients:** Chicken breast, spinach, feta cheese, garlic, olive oil, salt, and pepper.
- **Instructions**: Butterfly chicken breast. Sauté spinach and garlic in olive oil. Stuff chicken breast with spinach and feta mixture. Bake until chicken is cooked through.

Black Bean and Vegetable Quesadillas

- **Ingredients**: Whole grain tortillas, black beans, bell peppers, onions, corn, low-fat cheese, olive oil.
- **Instructions**: Sauté vegetables in olive oil until tender. Lay out tortillas, spread black beans, add sautéed vegetables and cheese. Fold tortillas in half and cook until the cheese is melted.

Salmon and Vegetable Foil Packets

- **Ingredients:** Salmon filets, bell peppers, zucchini, cherry tomatoes, olive oil, lemon juice, garlic, salt, and pepper.
- **Instructions**: Place salmon and vegetables on a piece of foil. Drizzle with olive oil, lemon juice, garlic, salt, and pepper. Seal foil packets and bake until salmon is cooked.

Mediterranean Chickpea Salad

- **Ingredients**: Chickpeas, cucumber, cherry tomatoes, red onion, olives, feta cheese, olive oil, lemon juice, garlic, salt, and pepper.
- **Instructions**: Mix all ingredients together in a bowl. Drizzle with olive oil and lemon juice. Season with garlic, salt, and pepper.

Vegetable and Lentil Soup:

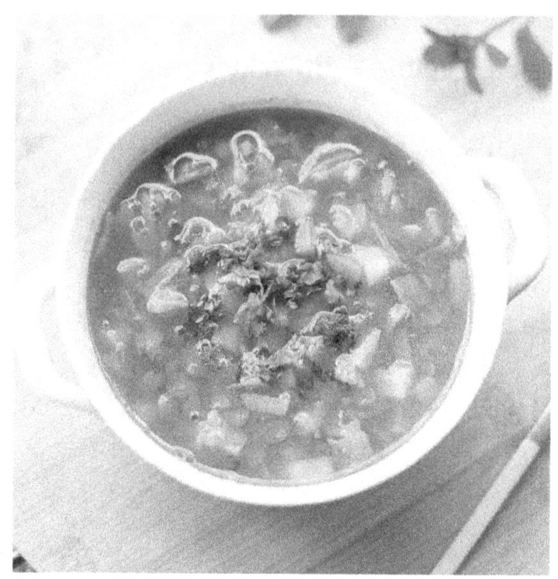

- **Ingredients**: Lentils, carrots, celery, onion, garlic, low-sodium vegetable broth, spinach, olive oil, salt, and pepper.
- **Instructions**: Sauté onions, carrots, celery, and garlic in olive oil until softened. Add lentils and vegetable broth. Simmer until lentils are cooked. Add the spinach and season with pepper and salt.

These recipes are not only delicious but also diabetic-friendly, providing balanced nutrition without causing spikes in blood sugar levels.

Snack

Greek Yogurt Parfait

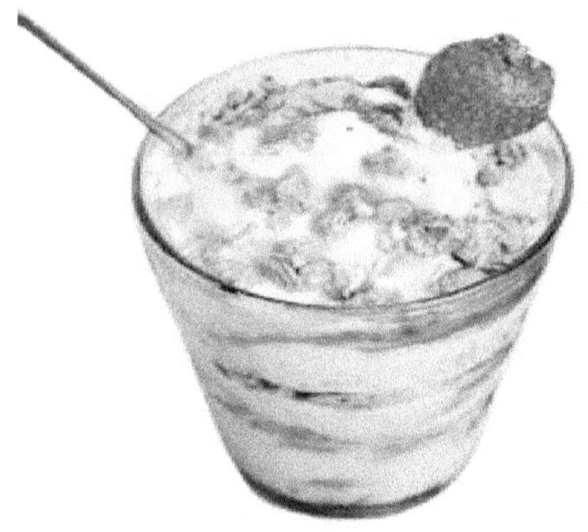

Ingredients:

- Greek yogurt (unsweetened)
- Berries (e.g., strawberries, blueberries)
- Nuts (e.g., almonds, walnuts)
- Cinnamon (optional)

Preparation:

- In a bowl or glass, layer Greek yogurt with berries.

- If preferred, top with a small amount of cinnamon and a sprinkle of nuts.
- Repeat layers as desired.

Nutritional Benefits:
- Greek yogurt provides protein and probiotics, berries offer antioxidants and fiber, while nuts supply healthy fats and additional protein.

Veggie Sticks with Hummus

Ingredients:
- Carrot sticks
- Cucumber sticks
- Bell pepper strips
- Hummus (store-bought or homemade)

Preparation:
- Wash and cut vegetables into sticks or strips.
- Serve with a side of hummus for dipping.

Nutritional Benefits:
- Colorful vegetables provide vitamins, minerals, and fiber, while hummus offers protein and healthy fats.

Apple Slices with Peanut Butter

Ingredients:

- Apple slices
- Natural peanut butter (unsweetened)

Preparation:

- Slice apples into wedges or rounds.Spread peanut butter on each apple slice.

Nutritional Benefits:

- Apples provide fiber and antioxidants, while natural peanut butter offers protein and healthy fats.

Cottage Cheese with Cherry Tomatoes

Ingredients:

- Cottage cheese (low-fat or non-fat)Cherry tomatoes
- Fresh basil leaves (optional)

Preparation:

- Spoon cottage cheese into a bowl.
- Halve cherry tomatoes and add them on top.
- Garnish with fresh basil leaves if desired.

Nutritional Benefits:

- Cottage cheese is a good source of protein and calcium, while cherry tomatoes provide vitamins and antioxidants.

Whole Grain Crackers with Avocado

Ingredients:
- Whole grain crackers
- Ripe avocado
- Lemon juice (optional)
- Red pepper flakes (optional)

Preparation:
- Mash ripe avocado in a bowl and season with lemon juice and red pepper flakes if desired.
- Spread avocado mixture on whole grain crackers.

Nutritional Benefits:
- Whole grain crackers offer fiber, while avocado provides healthy fats, vitamins, and minerals.

Hard-Boiled Eggs with Sliced Cucumber

Ingredients:
- Hard-boiled eggs
- Cucumber, sliced
- Everything bagel seasoning (optional)

Preparation:
- Hard-boiled eggs should be peeled and cut in half.
- Serve with sliced cucumber and sprinkle with everything bagel seasoning if desired.

Nutritional Benefits:
- Hard-boiled eggs are rich in protein and vitamins, while cucumber offers hydration and vitamins.

Trail Mix with Nuts and Seeds

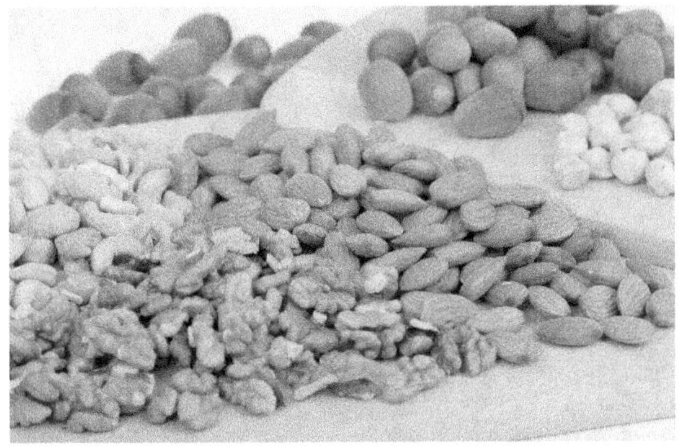

Ingredients:

- Mixed nuts (e.g., almonds, cashews, peanuts)
- Pumpkin seeds
- Sunflower seeds
- Dried fruit (unsweetened, in moderation)

Preparation:

- Mix together nuts, seeds, and dried fruit in a bowl.
- Portion out into small snack bags for easy grab-and-go options.

Nutritional Benefits: Nuts and seeds provide healthy fats, protein, and fiber, while dried fruit offers natural sweetness and additional nutrients.

Vegetable Sushi Rolls

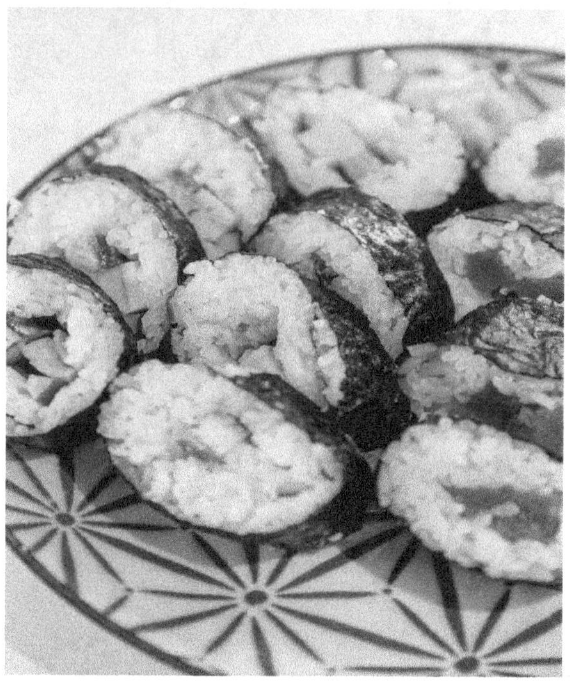

Ingredients:
- Nori seaweed sheets
- Cooked brown rice
- Assorted vegetables (e.g., cucumber, avocado, carrot, bell pepper)
- Soy sauce (low-sodium)

Preparation:

- Place a nori sheet on a clean surface and spread a thin layer of cooked brown rice.
- Arrange thinly sliced vegetables in the center of the nori sheet.
- Roll tightly and slice into bite-sized pieces.

Serve with low-sodium soy sauce for dipping.
Nutritional Benefits: Nori seaweed provides minerals, while brown rice and vegetables offer fiber, vitamins, and antioxidants.

Baked Sweet Potato Fries

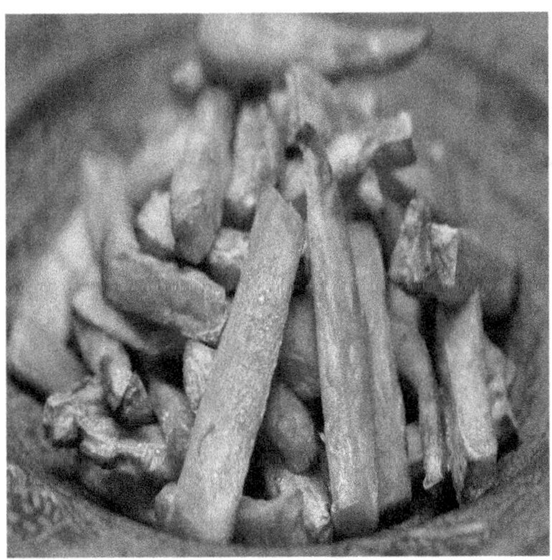

Ingredients:

- Sweet potatoes
- Olive Oil
- Paprika
- Garlic powder

Preparation:

- Preheat the oven to 425°F (220°C).
- Cut sweet potatoes into fries and toss with olive oil, paprika, and garlic powder.
- Place fries on a parchment paper-lined baking sheet.
- Bake until crispy, stirring halfway through, 25 to 30 minutes.

Nutritional Benefits: Sweet potatoes offer fiber, vitamins, and antioxidants, while olive oil provides healthy fats.

Chia Seed Pudding with Berries

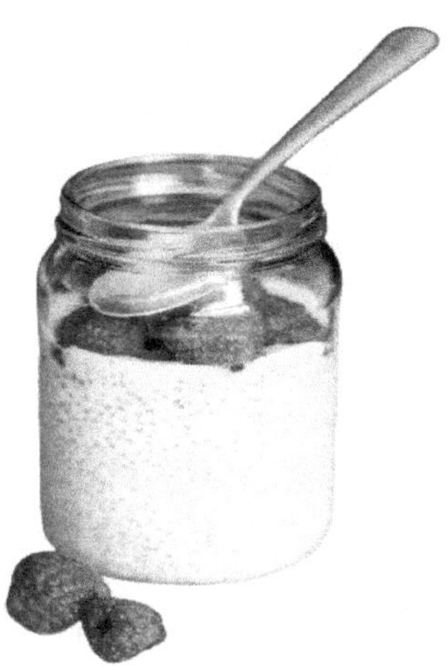

Ingredients:
- Chia Seeds
- Almond milk without sugar (or any other type of milk)
- Berries (e.g., strawberries, raspberries, blueberries)
- Vanilla extract (optional)
- Stevia or monk fruit sweetener (optional)

Preparation:

- Mix chia seeds with almond milk and vanilla extract in a bowl.
- If desired, sweeten with stevia or monk fruit sweetener.
- Refrigerate for at least 2 hours or overnight until pudding consistency forms.Serve with fresh berries on top.

Nutritional Benefits:

- Chia seeds are rich in fiber and omega-3 fatty acids, almond milk provides calcium and vitamin E, while berries offer antioxidants and fiber.

Dinner Recipes for Diabetics

Grilled Lemon Herb Chicken with Steamed Vegetables

Ingredients:
- Chicken breasts
- Lemon juice
- Olive oil
- Garlic
- Mixed herbs (e.g., rosemary, thyme)
- Assorted vegetables (e.g., broccoli, carrots, cauliflower)

Preparation:
- Marinate chicken breasts in lemon juice, olive oil, minced garlic, and mixed herbs for 30 minutes.
- Grill chicken until cooked through.
- Steam assorted vegetables until tender.

Health Benefits:
- Chicken is a lean source of protein, lemon juice adds flavor without added sugar, olive oil provides healthy fats, and vegetables offer vitamins, minerals, and fiber.

Salmon with Roasted Brussels Sprouts and Quinoa

Ingredients:
- Salmon filets
- Brussels sprouts
- Olive oil
- Garlic powder
- Quinoa

Preparation:
- Preheat the oven to 400°F (200°C).
- Toss Brussels sprouts with olive oil and garlic powder, then roast until tender.
- Season salmon filets with salt and pepper, then bake until cooked through.
- Cook quinoa according to package instructions.

Health Benefits:
- Salmon provides omega-3 fatty acids, Brussels sprouts offer fiber and vitamins, quinoa is a whole grain rich in protein and fiber.

Vegetable Stir-Fry with Tofu and Brown Rice

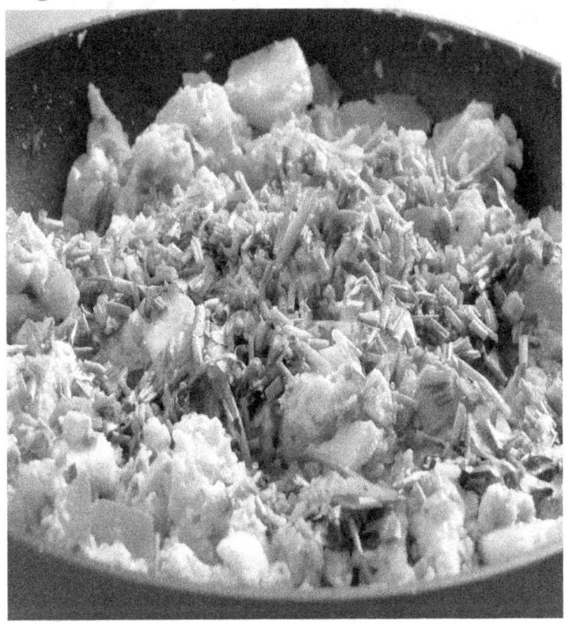

Ingredients:

- Tofu
- Various vegetables, such as broccoli, snap peas, and bell peppers
- Soy sauce (low-sodium)
- Garlic
- Ginger
- Brown rice

Preparation:

- Press tofu to remove excess moisture, then dice into cubes.
- Stir-fry tofu in a pan until golden brown, then set aside.
- Stir-fry assorted vegetables with minced garlic and ginger until tender-crisp.
- Add tofu back to the pan, then drizzle with low-sodium soy sauce.
- Serve with cooked brown rice.

Health Benefits:

- Tofu provides plant-based protein, vegetables offer fiber and vitamins, brown rice is a whole grain rich in fiber.

Turkey and Vegetable Quinoa Bowl

Ingredients:

- Ground turkey
- Quinoa
- Assorted vegetables (e.g., bell peppers, zucchini, carrots)
- Olive oil
- Italian seasoning

Preparation:

- Cook the ground turkey in a skillet until it's nicely browned.
- Cook quinoa according to package instructions.
- Stir-fry assorted vegetables in olive oil and Italian seasoning until tender.
- Assemble quinoa bowls with turkey, vegetables, and optional toppings like avocado or feta cheese.

Health Benefits:

- Ground turkey is lean protein, quinoa is a whole grain rich in protein and fiber, vegetables offer vitamins, minerals, and fiber.

Eggplant Parmesan with Whole Wheat Pasta

Ingredients:

- Eggplant
- Whole wheat pasta
- Tomato sauce (unsweetened)
- Mozzarella cheese
- Parmesan cheese

Preparation:
- Cut eggplant into rounds and roast it until it becomes soft.
- Use the package guidelines to cook the whole wheat pasta to perfection.
- Layer eggplant slices with tomato sauce and cheeses, then bake until bubbly.
- Serve with cooked whole wheat pasta.

Health Benefits:
- Eggplant is low in calories and carbohydrates, whole wheat pasta provides fiber and complex carbohydrates, tomato sauce offers antioxidants.

Lentil and Vegetable Curry with Brown Rice

Ingredients:
- Lentils
- Assorted vegetables (e.g., spinach, carrots, bell peppers)
- Coconut milk (light)
- Curry paste or powder
- Brown rice

Preparation:

- Cook lentils according to package instructions.
- Stir-fry assorted vegetables in a pot, then add cooked lentils, coconut milk, and curry paste or powder.
- Simmer until vegetables are tender and flavors are well-combined.
- Serve over cooked brown rice.

Health Benefits:

- Lentils are rich in fiber and protein, vegetables offer vitamins and minerals, brown rice provides fiber and complex carbohydrates.

Grilled Shrimp and Vegetable Skewers with Quinoa:

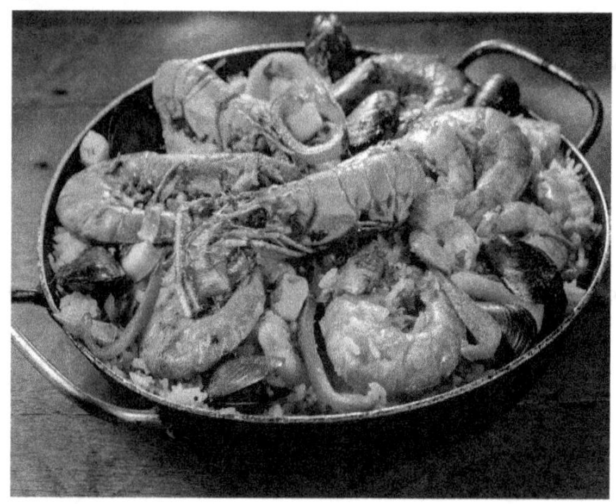

Ingredients:

- Shrimp
- Assorted vegetables (e.g., cherry tomatoes, bell peppers, zucchini)
- Olive oil
- Lemon juice
- Quinoa

Preparation:
- Marinate shrimp in olive oil and lemon juice, then thread onto skewers with assorted vegetables.
- Grill skewers until shrimp are pink and vegetables are tender.
- Cook quinoa according to package instructions.

Health Benefits:
- Shrimp is low in calories and high in protein, vegetables offer fiber and vitamins, quinoa is a whole grain rich in protein and fiber.

Baked Chicken Breast with Roasted Root Vegetables:

Ingredients:
- Chicken breast
- Assorted root vegetables (e.g., carrots, sweet potatoes, parsnips)
- Olive oil
- Garlic powder
- Thyme

Preparation:

- Season chicken breasts with garlic powder, thyme, salt, and pepper.
- Arrange chicken and assorted root vegetables on a baking sheet.
- Drizzle with olive oil and roast until chicken is cooked through and vegetables are tender.

Health Benefits:

- Chicken is lean protein, root vegetables offer vitamins and minerals, olive oil provides healthy fats.

Turkey and Bean Chili:

Ingredients:
- Ground turkey
- Kidney beans
- Black beans
- Tomato sauce (unsweetened)
- Bell peppers
- Onion
- Chili powder

Preparation:
- Brown ground turkey in a pot, then add chopped bell peppers and onion.Stir in kidney beans, black beans, tomato sauce, and chili powder.Simmer until flavors are well-combined and chili is heated through.

Health Benefits:
- Ground turkey is lean protein, beans offer fiber and protein, bell peppers are rich in vitamins and antioxidants.

Importance of Diet for Diabetic Patients

In the battle against diabetes, diet plays a pivotal role in blood sugar control and overall management. A balanced and personalized eating plan designed to individual needs can make all the difference in maintaining stable blood sugar levels, preventing complications, and improving overall health.

Diet directly impacts blood sugar levels, making it a cornerstone of diabetes management. Since carbohydrates are converted to sugar during digestion, they specifically have the biggest impact on blood glucose levels. Controlling carbohydrate intake, along with balancing it with protein, fat, and fiber, can help regulate blood sugar levels throughout the day. Moreover, dietary choices influence weight management, insulin sensitivity, and the risk of developing complications associated with diabetes.

Impact of Diet on Long-Term Complications and Health

Following a balanced and personalized eating plan can significantly reduce the risk of long-term complications associated with diabetes, such as heart disease, kidney disease, nerve damage, and vision problems. By maintaining stable blood sugar levels and supporting overall health through dietary choices, individuals with diabetes can enjoy a higher quality of life and better manage their condition in the long run.

In summary, diet plays a critical role in managing diabetes and promoting overall health. By focusing on whole, unprocessed foods, fiber-rich choices, lean proteins, healthy fats, and low-glycemic index foods, individuals can effectively control blood sugar levels, reduce the risk of complications, and improve their well-being. Consulting a registered dietitian or healthcare provider for personalized guidance and support is key to developing a sustainable and effective eating plan for diabetes management.

CHAPTER FIVE

Smart Food Choices for Diabetes Management

Foods for Diabetes Management:

Leafy Greens: Rich in vitamins, minerals, and antioxidants are spinach, kale, and Swiss chard. They're low in calories and carbohydrates, making them excellent choices for managing blood sugar levels.

Berries: Blueberries, strawberries, and raspberries are rich in fiber, vitamins, and antioxidants. They have a low glycemic index, meaning they won't cause spikes in blood sugar levels.

Nuts and Seeds: Almonds, walnuts, flaxseeds, and chia seeds are high in healthy fats, protein, and fiber. They help keep you full, stabilize blood sugar levels, and improve heart health.

Fatty Fish: Salmon, mackerel, and sardines are rich in omega-3 fatty acids, which have anti-inflammatory properties and support heart health. Try to get two or more servings of fatty fish per week.

Sweet Potatoes: Rich in fiber, vitamins, and minerals, sweet potatoes have a lower glycemic index than regular potatoes. They provide sustained energy without causing rapid spikes in blood sugar levels.

Avocados: Full of monounsaturated fats, avocados help improve insulin sensitivity and lower cholesterol levels. They're also rich in fiber and potassium, which are beneficial for heart health.

Legumes: Beans, lentils, and chickpeas are high in fiber and protein, making them excellent choices for managing blood sugar levels and promoting satiety.

Whole Grains: Oats, quinoa, and barley are rich in fiber, vitamins, and minerals. They help stabilize blood sugar levels, improve digestion, and reduce the risk of heart disease.

Herbs and Spices: Cinnamon, turmeric, and ginger have been shown to improve insulin sensitivity and reduce inflammation. They can be used to add flavor to dishes without adding extra calories or sugar.

Non-Starchy Vegetables: Broccoli, cauliflower, peppers, and cucumbers are low in calories and carbohydrates but high in fiber and nutrients. They're great for filling up your plate without spiking blood sugar levels.

Meal Planning and Grocery Shopping Tips:

Reading Food Labels: Look for foods low in added sugars, saturated fats, and sodium. Pay attention to portion sizes and aim for products with whole ingredients.

Identifying Healthy Fats and Protein Sources:
Choose lean proteins like chicken, turkey, and tofu,
and options for sources of healthy fats like olive oil,
avocado, and nuts.

Choosing Whole Grains and Fiber-Rich Foods:
Option for whole grains like brown rice, quinoa,
and whole wheat bread, and include plenty of fruits,
vegetables, and legumes in your diet for added fiber.

Avoiding Added Sugars and Refined Carbs:
Minimize intake of sugary beverages, desserts, and
processed foods, which can cause rapid spikes in
blood sugar levels.

Healthy Eating Habits:

Eating Regular, Balanced Meals: Aim for three
meals a day, with healthy snacks if needed. Include
a balance of carbohydrates, protein, and healthy fats
in each meal to help regulate blood sugar levels.

Incorporating Physical Activity into Daily Routine: Stay active with regular exercise, such as walking, swimming, or yoga. Physical activity helps improve insulin sensitivity and promotes overall health and well-being.

Staying Hydrated: Drink plenty of water throughout the day to stay hydrated and support optimal body function. Limit sugary beverages and options for water, herbal tea, or sparkling water instead.

Managing Portion Sizes: Use measuring cups, spoons, or visual cues to control portion sizes and avoid overeating. Focus on eating slowly and mindfully, paying attention to hunger and fullness cues.

You may effectively control your diabetes and enhance your general health and well-being by adopting these wise food choices and good eating habits into your daily routine. For individualized advice and support, don't forget to speak with a licensed dietician or healthcare professional.

Fruits and Vegetables for Diabetics

Maintaining a balanced diet is essential for managing diabetes, especially as we age. Among the plethora of food choices, fruits and vegetables stand out as indispensable allies in the battle against fluctuating blood sugar levels. Here's why:

Nature's Bounty: Fruits and vegetables offer a treasure trove of nutrients vital for overall health, including vitamins, minerals, antioxidants, and fiber. These nutrients play pivotal roles in regulating blood sugar levels, improving insulin sensitivity, and reducing the risk of diabetes-related complications.

Fiber: A Diabetic's Best Friend: Fiber is particularly beneficial for individuals with diabetes. Soluble fiber, found abundantly in fruits like berries, apples, and oranges, slows down digestion and the absorption of carbohydrates, preventing sudden spikes in blood sugar levels. Meanwhile, insoluble fiber, prevalent in vegetables like broccoli, Brussels sprouts, and cauliflower, promotes digestive health and helps maintain steady blood sugar levels.

Antioxidants to the Rescue: Many fruits and vegetables are rich in antioxidants, such as vitamin C, vitamin E, and beta-carotene. These compounds help combat inflammation and oxidative stress, which are common culprits in diabetes and its complications. Berries, spinach, kale, and bell peppers are among the top contenders in the antioxidant-rich category.

Low Glycemic Index Champions: Certain fruits and vegetables have a low glycemic index (GI), meaning they cause a gradual rise in blood sugar levels. They are therefore the best options for those who have diabetes. Examples include leafy greens like spinach and kale, cruciferous vegetables like broccoli and cauliflower, and citrus fruits like oranges.

Mindful Choices: While fruits are generally healthy, it's crucial for individuals with diabetes to be mindful of their portion sizes and the glycemic load of the fruits they consume. Opting for whole fruits over juices and incorporating a variety of colorful fruits and vegetables into meals ensures a diverse array of nutrients and flavors.

Fruit and Vegetables

Spinach: Rich in iron, calcium, and vitamins A and C, spinach is low in carbohydrates and calories. Its high fiber content aids in blood sugar control and promotes heart health.

Broccoli: Packed with antioxidants, including vitamin C and beta-carotene, broccoli helps lower blood sugar levels and reduces insulin resistance. It's also high in fiber, promoting digestive health.

Berries (e.g., Blueberries, Strawberries, Raspberries): These fruits are low in sugar and high in fiber and antioxidants, such as anthocyanins, which help improve insulin sensitivity and lower inflammation.

Avocado: Although technically a fruit, avocados are low in carbohydrates and high in healthy fats, particularly monounsaturated fats, which can improve insulin sensitivity. They also provide fiber and potassium.

Brussels Sprouts: Packed with fiber, vitamins, and minerals, Brussels sprouts have a low glycemic index, making them an excellent choice for managing blood sugar levels and promoting satiety.

Oranges: Despite their sweet taste, oranges are low in calories and high in fiber and vitamin C. The soluble fiber in oranges helps slow glucose absorption, preventing blood sugar spikes.

Cauliflower: Low in carbohydrates and calories, cauliflower is rich in fiber, vitamins, and antioxidants. It can support weight control and enhance insulin sensitivity.

Apples: High in fiber and antioxidants, such as quercetin, apples can help stabilize blood sugar levels and reduce the risk of diabetes complications. Eating the whole fruit, including the skin, maximizes its nutritional benefits.

Kale: Packed with vitamins A, C, and K, as well as antioxidants and fiber, kale supports blood sugar control and heart health. Its low calorie and carbohydrate content make it an ideal choice for diabetics.

Bell Peppers: Rich in vitamins A and C, bell peppers are low in carbohydrates and calories. Their high fiber content helps regulate blood sugar levels, while their antioxidants combat inflammation and oxidative stress.

Lean Protein Sources and Plant-Based Alternatives

Including plant-based substitutes and lean protein sources can help control blood sugar levels and enhance general health.

Lean Protein Sources:

Skinless Poultry: Chicken and turkey breast are excellent sources of lean protein. They are low in saturated fat, making them ideal choices for individuals with diabetes.

Fish: Fatty fish like salmon, mackerel, and sardines are rich in omega-3 fatty acids, which have been shown to improve heart health and reduce inflammation. Fish is a healthful food whether grilled or baked.

Eggs: An inexpensive and adaptable source of protein are eggs. Research suggests that consuming eggs in moderation does not adversely affect blood sugar levels and may even improve satiety.

Lean Cuts of Meat: Option for lean cuts of beef and pork, such as sirloin and tenderloin. Trim visible fat before cooking to reduce saturated fat intake.

Legumes: Beans, lentils, and chickpeas are high in protein and fiber, making them excellent choices for stabilizing blood sugar levels. They also contain complex carbohydrates that are digested more slowly, preventing rapid spikes in blood glucose.

Plant-Based Alternatives:

Tofu and Tempeh: These soy-based products are rich in protein and can be used as meat substitutes in various dishes. They are also low in saturated fat and cholesterol, making them heart-healthy options.

Quinoa: Quinoa is a complete protein, meaning it contains all nine essential amino acids. It is also a good source of fiber and has a low glycemic index, making it suitable for diabetes management.

Nuts and Seeds: Almonds, walnuts, chia seeds, and flaxseeds are nutritious plant-based sources of protein, healthy fats, and fiber. Incorporating them into meals or snacks can help control hunger and regulate blood sugar levels.

Legumes: In addition to being a lean protein source, legumes also provide essential nutrients like iron, magnesium, and potassium. They can be used in salads, soups, stews, and stir-fries for a satisfying and nutritious meal.

Vegetables: Some vegetables, such as broccoli, spinach, and Brussels sprouts, contain significant amounts of protein. Including a variety of vegetables in your diet not only provides essential nutrients but also helps control calorie intake and manage weight.

Healthy Fats and Oils

Those with diabetes must maintain a balanced diet, particularly as they get older. Including heart-healthy fats and oils in the diet can help lower blood sugar, promote overall well being, and strengthen the heart.

Here are some healthy fats and oils to consider:
Olive Oil: Olive oil is rich in monounsaturated fats, which have been linked to numerous health benefits, including improved insulin sensitivity and lower risk of heart disease. Use extra virgin olive oil for salads and low-temperature cooking, and regular olive oil for sautéing and baking.

Avocado: Avocados are packed with monounsaturated fats, fiber, and various vitamins and minerals. They can be enjoyed sliced on toast, blended into smoothies, or used as a creamy substitute for mayonnaise in sandwiches and salads.

Nuts and Seeds: Almonds, walnuts, flaxseeds, chia seeds, and pumpkin seeds are excellent sources of healthy fats, protein, and fiber. Snack on a handful of nuts or sprinkle seeds on salads, yogurt, or oatmeal for added crunch and nutrition.

Fatty Fish: Salmon, mackerel, trout, and sardines are rich in omega-3 fatty acids, which are beneficial for heart health and reducing inflammation. Aim to include fatty fish in your diet at least twice a week to reap the health benefits.

Flaxseed Oil: Flaxseed oil is a plant-based source of omega-3 fatty acids, particularly alpha-linolenic acid (ALA). It can be drizzled over salads or added to smoothies for a nutritional boost. Store flaxseed oil in the refrigerator to prevent it from going rancid.

Canola Oil: Canola oil is low in saturated fat and rich in heart-healthy monounsaturated fats. It has a neutral flavor, making it suitable for both cooking and baking. Look for cold-pressed or expeller-pressed canola oil for the highest quality.

Nut Butter: Peanut butter, almond butter, and cashew butter are delicious spreads that provide healthy fats, protein, and fiber. Choose natural nut butters without added sugars or hydrogenated oils for the best nutritional value.

CHAPTER SIX

Strategies for Dining Out and Social Events

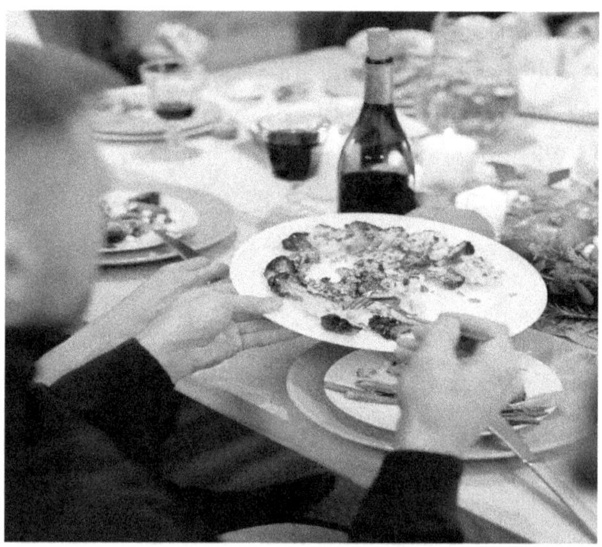

Dining out and attending social events can present challenges, but with the right strategies, managing blood sugar levels can remain achievable and enjoyable.

Plan Ahead: Research the restaurant's menu online in advance to identify healthier options and portion sizes. Many establishments now offer nutritional information, making it easier to make informed choices.

Choose Wisely: Option for dishes that are grilled, steamed, baked, or broiled instead of fried. Look for lean protein sources like grilled chicken or fish, and prioritize vegetables and whole grains. Avoid dishes with excessive sauces, creams, or added sugars.

Portion Control: Pay attention to portion sizes, which can often be larger than necessary. Try asking for a smaller serving or splitting the meal with someone. As an alternative, you can get a box to go and pack away half of your meal before you even begin to eat.

Mindful Eating: Eat slowly and savor each bite. This allows time for your body to register fullness, helping to prevent overeating. Engage in conversation and focus on enjoying the company rather than solely on the food.

Stay Hydrated: Drink water throughout the meal to stay hydrated and to help control your appetite. Avoid sugary drinks and excessive alcohol, as they can cause spikes in blood sugar levels.

Be Assertive: Don't hesitate to communicate your dietary needs to the server. Most restaurants are willing to accommodate special requests, such as substituting sides or preparing dishes without certain ingredients.

Navigate the Buffet: When faced with a buffet, survey all options before filling your plate. Start with a salad or vegetables, then add lean proteins and whole grains. Limit your intake of high-carb or sugary items like bread, pasta, and desserts.

Manage Temptations: If desserts are offered, consider sharing with others or opting for a fruit-based option. Alternatively, satisfy your sweet tooth with a small piece of dark chocolate or a few berries.

Check Blood Sugar Levels: Monitor your blood sugar levels before and after dining out to gauge the impact of your meal choices. This can help you learn how different foods affect your body and adjust your eating habits accordingly.

Stay Active: Incorporate physical activity into your routine, both before and after dining out. A short walk after a meal can help lower blood sugar levels and aid digestion.

By putting these tips into practice, people with diabetes over 50 can eat great meals while controlling their blood sugar levels, and they can even enjoy dining out and social gatherings with confidence. Recall that the secret to long-term success in managing diabetes is moderation and consistency.

Tips for Navigating Restaurant Menus

Eating out can be a challenge for anyone trying to maintain a diabetic diet, especially as we age. However, with a few simple strategies, navigating restaurant menus can become easier and more enjoyable while still adhering to dietary restrictions.

Plan Ahead: Before heading to a restaurant, check the menu online if possible. Look for healthier options such as grilled or baked dishes, salads, and steamed vegetables. Planning ahead allows you to make informed choices rather than feeling pressured in the moment.

Portion Control: Restaurant portions are often much larger than what is recommended for a diabetic diet. Consider sharing a meal with a dining partner or ask for a to-go box to portion out half of your meal before you start eating. This helps control calorie intake and prevents overeating.

Choose Wisely: Option for dishes that are grilled, baked, or steamed instead of fried or sautéed. Look for lean protein sources like chicken, fish, or tofu, and ask for sauces and dressings on the side to control the amount you consume.

Watch Your Carbs: Be mindful of carbohydrate-rich foods like bread, pasta, rice, and potatoes. Instead, choose whole grains when available and substitute side dishes with extra servings of vegetables or a salad.

Beware of Hidden Sugars: Many restaurant dishes contain hidden sugars in sauces, marinades, and dressings. Ask about the ingredients or request these items on the side so you can control how much you consume.

Stay Hydrated: Drink water or other non-caloric beverages instead of sugary drinks like soda or fruit juice. Limit alcohol consumption, as it can affect blood sugar levels and interact with diabetes medications.

Don't Be Afraid to Customize: Don't hesitate to ask for substitutions or modifications to better fit your dietary needs. Most restaurants are willing to accommodate special requests, such as replacing fries with a side salad or skipping the breadbasket.

Practice Mindful Eating: Take your time to savor each bite and listen to your body's hunger and fullness cues. You can avoid overindulging and savor your food to the fullest by eating gently.

Ask for Nutritional Information: Some restaurants provide nutritional information for their menu items upon request. Use this information to make informed choices that align with your dietary goals.

Be Prepared for Social Situations: Dining out with friends and family can sometimes lead to pressure to indulge in unhealthy foods. Be confident in your choices and politely explain your dietary restrictions if necessary. Give more thought to the discussion and company than just the food.

Managing Blood Sugar During Special Occasions

Preventing blood sugar rises and preserving general health primarily involves eating a balanced diet and making thoughtful decisions. For diabetics over 50, this guide offers tips and tactics for managing special occasions without compromising blood sugar control.

Plan Ahead:
- Before attending a special occasion, plan your meals and snacks to ensure they align with your dietary needs and blood sugar goals.
- Consider eating a balanced meal or snack before the event to prevent overindulging in high-carb or sugary foods later.

Monitor Portion Sizes:
- Be mindful of portion sizes, especially when faced with tempting foods that may affect blood sugar levels.
- Use smaller plates to control portion sizes and avoid overeating.

Choose Wisely:
- Option for healthier food options such as vegetables, lean proteins, and whole grains.
- Limit intake of high-carb and high-sugar foods like desserts, sugary beverages, and refined carbohydrates.
- If dessert is a must, choose smaller portions and opt for fruit-based desserts or those made with sugar substitutes.

Stay Hydrated:
- Drink plenty of water throughout the event to stay hydrated and help control appetite.
- Limit alcohol consumption, as it can affect blood sugar levels and lead to overeating.

Be Mindful of Timing:
- Pay attention to meal timings and spacing to prevent prolonged periods of high or low blood sugar.
- If meals are delayed, have a healthy snack to prevent hypoglycemia.

Monitor Blood Sugar Levels:
- Regularly monitor blood sugar levels before, during, and after the event to gauge the impact of food choices and adjust insulin or medication doses if necessary.

Stay Active:
- Incorporate physical activity into your routine, even during special occasions. Take short walks or engage in light exercises to help manage blood sugar levels.

Communicate with Hosts:
- Inform hosts or caterers about your dietary needs and preferences, especially if you have specific dietary restrictions due to diabetes.

Alcohol and Diabetes: Guidelines for Consumption

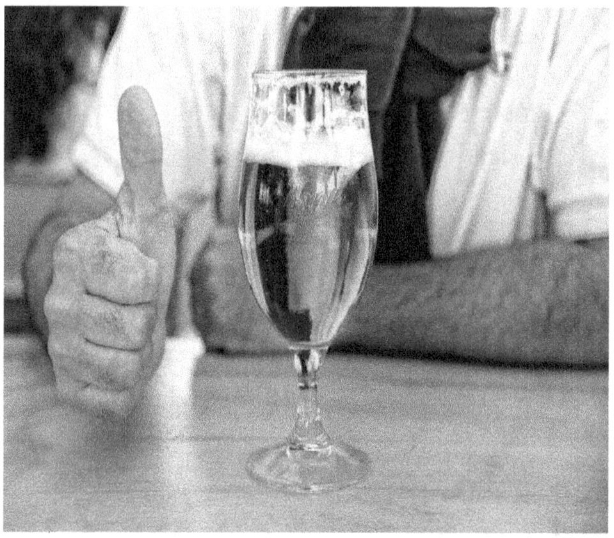

For individuals over 50 with diabetes, understanding the effects of alcohol on blood sugar levels is crucial for maintaining optimal health. While moderate alcohol consumption may have certain benefits, it can also pose risks for those managing diabetes.

Understand the Effects of Alcohol:

- Alcohol can affect blood sugar levels both immediately and in the hours following consumption.
- It may initially cause blood sugar levels to rise due to the carbohydrates present in certain alcoholic beverages.
- However, excessive alcohol consumption can lead to hypoglycemia (low blood sugar) hours later, especially for individuals taking insulin or certain diabetes medications.

Limit Consumption:

- Moderate alcohol consumption is generally considered safe for most individuals with diabetes.
- Men should not consume more than two drinks of alcohol in a day, while women should only have one drink.
- One drink is typically defined as 12 ounces of beer, 5 ounces of wine, or 1.5 ounces of distilled spirits.

Choose Wisely:

- Option for alcoholic beverages that are lower in sugar and carbohydrates to minimize their impact on blood sugar levels.
- Dry wines, light beers, and distilled spirits with low-carb mixers are generally better choices than sweetened cocktails or sugary mixed drinks.

Monitor Blood Sugar Levels:
- Regularly monitor blood sugar levels before and after consuming alcohol to understand its effects on your body.
- Be prepared to treat any fluctuations in blood sugar levels accordingly, especially if you are at risk of hypoglycemia.

Eat Before Drinking:
- Consuming food before drinking can help slow down the absorption of alcohol into the bloodstream and mitigate its impact on blood sugar levels.
- Choose balanced meals or snacks that include carbohydrates, protein, and healthy fats to help stabilize blood sugar levels.

Stay Hydrated:

- Drink plenty of water while consuming alcohol to stay hydrated and prevent dehydration, which can exacerbate fluctuations in blood sugar levels.

Be Cautious with Medications:

- Some diabetes medications, particularly those that stimulate insulin production or increase insulin sensitivity, can interact with alcohol and increase the risk of hypoglycemia.
- Consult with your healthcare provider to understand how alcohol may interact with your specific medications and adjust your treatment plan accordingly.

Know When to Avoid Alcohol:
- There are certain situations in which individuals with diabetes should avoid alcohol altogether, such as when blood sugar levels are not well-controlled or during periods of illness or medication adjustments.
- Pregnant women with diabetes should also abstain from alcohol to prevent potential harm to the fetus.

In summary, moderate alcohol consumption can be a part of a balanced lifestyle for individuals over 50 with diabetes, but it requires careful consideration and monitoring. By understanding the effects of alcohol on blood sugar levels and following these guidelines for responsible consumption, diabetics can enjoy alcohol in moderation while maintaining optimal health. As always, consult with a healthcare provider for personalized advice based on individual health needs and medication regimens.

CHAPTER SEVEN

The Role of Exercise in Diabetes Management

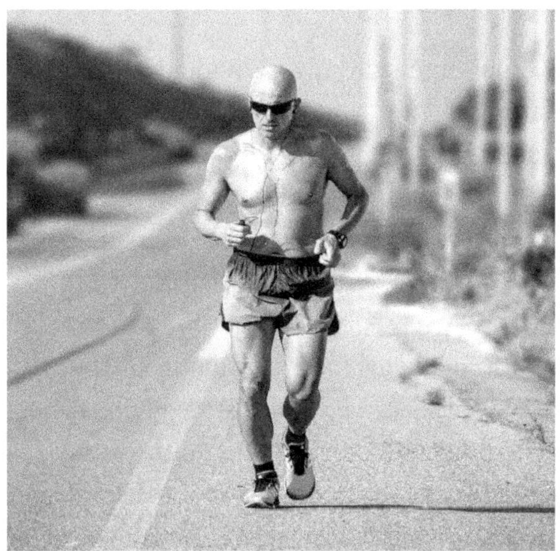

Exercise is essential for treating diabetes, particularly in people over 50. Here is a thorough analysis of its importance:

Blood Sugar Control: Exercise helps regulate blood sugar levels by increasing insulin sensitivity, allowing cells to use glucose more effectively. This reduces the need for insulin medication and can prevent complications associated with high blood sugar.

Weight Management: Many individuals with diabetes struggle with weight gain, which exacerbates insulin resistance. Regular exercise helps maintain a healthy weight or facilitates weight loss by burning calories and building lean muscle mass.

Heart Health: Diabetes increases the risk of cardiovascular diseases. Exercise strengthens the heart muscle, lowers blood pressure, improves circulation, and reduces the risk of heart disease and stroke.

Improvement in Lipid Profile: Physical activity can raise HDL (good) cholesterol levels and lower LDL (bad) cholesterol levels, reducing the risk of heart disease and stroke, common complications of diabetes.

Stress Reduction: Managing diabetes can be stressful, but exercise helps reduce stress levels by releasing endorphins, the body's natural mood elevators. This can positively impact overall mental well-being and enhance quality of life.

Enhanced Insulin Action: Exercise promotes glucose uptake by muscles, even in the absence of insulin, making it an essential component of diabetes management, particularly for those with type 2 diabetes who may have insulin resistance.

Prevention of Complications: Regular physical activity can help prevent or delay the onset of complications associated with diabetes, such as nerve damage, kidney disease, and eye problems, by improving overall health and reducing risk factors.

Improved Sleep Patterns: Diabetes can disrupt sleep patterns, leading to fatigue and exacerbating symptoms. Exercise promotes better sleep quality, aiding in overall health and diabetes management.

Social Engagement: Participating in group exercise classes or outdoor activities can foster social connections, reducing feelings of isolation and providing additional support for managing diabetes.

Individualized Approach: It's essential to tailor exercise plans to individual needs, considering factors such as age, fitness level, medical history, and any complications related to diabetes. Consulting with healthcare professionals or certified trainers can help develop safe and effective exercise routines.

In summary, exercise is a cornerstone of diabetes management, particularly for individuals over 50. Its benefits extend beyond blood sugar control to encompass overall health, well-being, and prevention of complications. Incorporating regular physical activity into daily life can significantly improve outcomes and quality of life for those living with diabetes.

Benefits of Physical Activity for Diabetics

Our bodies change as we get older, and these changes can have an effect on our general health, particularly for those who have diabetes. For diabetics over 50, regular physical exercise is essential since it provides a host of advantages that can help control the disease and enhance general health. This post will discuss the benefits of exercise for people with diabetes and offer advice on how to begin an activity program that is both safe and productive.

Benefits of Physical Activity for Diabetics:

- Improved Blood Sugar Control: Physical activity helps lower blood sugar levels and improve insulin sensitivity, reducing the risk of complications.
- Weight Management: Regular exercise aids in weight loss and maintenance, which is essential for managing diabetes.

- **Enhanced Insulin Sensitivity**: Physical activity improves the body's ability to use insulin, reducing the risk of developing insulin resistance.
- **Cardiovascular Health**: Exercise helps lower blood pressure, improve circulation, and reduce the risk of heart disease.
- **Increased Strength and Flexibility**: Regular physical activity helps build muscle mass and improve flexibility, reducing the risk of falls and injuries.
- **Better Mental Health**: Exercise has been shown to reduce stress, anxiety, and depression in individuals with diabetes.
- **Improved Sleep:** Regular physical activity can help improve sleep quality and duration.
- **Reduced Risk of Complications**: Physical activity has been shown to reduce the risk of diabetes-related complications, such as nerve damage and kidney disease.

Getting Started with Physical Activity:

1. **Consult Your Healthcare Provider:** Before starting any new exercise routine, consult with your healthcare provider to discuss any limitations or concerns.

2. **Choose Low-Impact Activities**: Option for low-impact activities like walking, swimming, or cycling, which are gentle on the joints.

3. **Start Slow**: Begin with short, manageable sessions (20-30 minutes) and gradually increase duration and intensity.

4. **Find an Exercise Buddy**: Having a workout partner can help keep you motivated and accountable.

5. **Mix it Up**: Incorporate a variety of activities to avoid boredom and prevent plateaus.

6. **Monitor Progress**: Keep track of your progress, including blood sugar levels, weight, and exercise routine.

Remember to listen to your body and rest when needed. It's essential to balance physical activity with proper nutrition and medication to manage your diabetes effectively.

Safe and Effective Exercises for Older Adults

Being physically active as we age is crucial for preserving our general health and wellbeing. But it's crucial to pick safe and efficient workouts, particularly for senior citizens. This is a thorough guide to safe and efficient exercise for senior citizens:

Walking: Make walking a daily habit to boost cardiovascular health, strengthen muscles, and maintain flexible joints. Most days of the week, try to get in at least 30 minutes of brisk walking.

Swimming is a great full-body exercise that is easy on the joints. It enhances flexibility, muscle strength, and cardiovascular fitness. For senior citizens, taking water aerobics programs or swimming laps are excellent choices.

Strength Training: Incorporating strength training exercises into your routine helps maintain muscle mass, bone density, and metabolism. Use resistance bands, free weights, or weight machines to perform exercises targeting major muscle groups, such as squats, lunges, chest presses, and rows. As strength increases, begin with lighter weights and progressively increase.

Tai Chi: Tai Chi is a gentle form of martial arts that focuses on slow, controlled movements and deep breathing. It improves balance, flexibility, and muscle strength while reducing stress and promoting relaxation. Tai Chi classes specifically designed for older adults are widely available and can be easily modified to accommodate different fitness levels.

Yoga: Yoga enhances flexibility, strength, and balance by combining physical postures, breathing techniques, and meditation. Additionally, it eases tension and encourages relaxation. Seek out gentle or chair yoga programs designed specifically for senior citizens; these can accommodate those with limited mobility or health difficulties.

Cycling: Cycling is a low-impact aerobic exercise that can be done outdoors or on a stationary bike. It improves cardiovascular health, leg strength, and joint mobility. Start with short rides at a comfortable pace and gradually increase duration and intensity.

Balance Exercises: Improving balance is crucial for preventing falls, especially as we age. Simple balance exercises like standing on one leg, heel-to-toe walking, and balance board exercises can help strengthen stabilizing muscles and improve coordination.

Flexibility Exercises: Stretching exercises help maintain joint flexibility and range of motion. Incorporate gentle stretching into your routine, focusing on major muscle groups such as hamstrings, calves, shoulders, and chest. Hold each stretch for 15-30 seconds without bouncing, and avoid stretching to the point of pain.

.

Pilates: Pilates is a great exercise for seniors, focusing on body awareness, flexibility, and core strength to improve balance and posture. Controlled movements and proper alignment help seniors stay stable and confident, with many studios offering senior-specific classes.

Consult a Professional: Before starting any new exercise program, especially if you have existing health concerns or medical conditions, consult with a healthcare professional or a certified fitness instructor. They can provide personalized recommendations and ensure you're engaging in activities that are safe and beneficial for your individual needs.

Older persons can maintain or increase their physical fitness, improve their quality of life, and lower their chance of developing age-related health problems by including a variety of these safe and efficient workouts into their daily routine. Always pay attention to your body, begin cautiously, and build up to a greater intensity and longer length over time. At any age, maintain an active lifestyle and reap the health advantages of consistent exercise.

Including Exercise in Everyday Routine

Including regular exercise into your daily routine is crucial for managing diabetes after the age of 50. Here's how you can seamlessly integrate physical activity into your life:

Morning Walks: Take a quick stroll to start your day. It not only increases metabolism but also aids in blood sugar regulation during the day.

Stair Climbing: Whenever feasible, choose the stairs over elevators. It's an easy, yet efficient, method to fit in a little additional exercise.

Home Workouts: Dedicate a corner of your home to simple workout routines like stretching, yoga, or light strength training. This allows you to exercise at your convenience, without the need for expensive equipment.

Dance Sessions: Put on your favorite tunes and dance around the house. Not only is it fun, but it's also a great cardiovascular workout that can help improve insulin sensitivity.

Active Hobbies: Engage in activities that you enjoy and that keep you moving, such as gardening, swimming, or cycling. These hobbies not only promote physical health but also provide mental relaxation.

Scheduled Breaks: If you have a desk job, make it a point to stand up and stretch every hour. Set reminders on your phone or computer to ensure you're not sitting for prolonged periods.

Evening Strolls: Wind down your day with a leisurely walk after dinner. It aids in digestion and helps lower post-meal blood sugar levels.

Group Activities: Start a walking club with friends or neighbors, or enroll in a nearby fitness class. Joining an exercise group can help with accountability and motivation.

Never forget to speak with your doctor before beginning a new fitness program, particularly if you have any underlying medical issues. After 50, you can maintain a healthier, more active lifestyle and effectively manage your diabetes by prioritizing physical activity in your daily routine.

CHAPTER EIGHT

Understanding Food Labels and Nutrition Facts

Knowing how to read food labels and comprehend nutrition information is essential for anyone managing diabetes, especially as they get older. This is a thorough guide on understanding food labels and selecting foods for a post-50 diabetes diet:

Serving Size Awareness: Start by examining the serving size listed on the nutrition label. This information dictates the portion size for which the nutritional content is provided. Be mindful of portion sizes to accurately assess the nutritional value of the food you consume.

Total Carbohydrates: Pay close attention to the total carbohydrate content, as carbohydrates have the most significant impact on blood sugar levels. Aim for foods with lower carbohydrate content per serving, and choose complex carbohydrates over simple sugars to help stabilize blood sugar levels.

Fiber Content: Look for foods high in dietary fiber, as fiber helps slow down the absorption of glucose and can aid in blood sugar control. Opt for whole grains, fruits, vegetables, legumes, and nuts, which are rich sources of fiber.

Sugars: Differentiate between naturally occurring sugars and added sugars on the nutrition label. While natural sugars found in fruits and dairy products are generally considered healthier options, added sugars should be limited, as they can contribute to spikes in blood sugar levels. Aim for foods with minimal added sugars or choose alternatives with no added sugars.

Protein and Fat: Consider the protein and fat content of foods, as they can influence satiety and blood sugar stability. Incorporate lean proteins and healthy fats into your diet, such as lean meats, fish, poultry, nuts, seeds, and avocado, while moderating intake of saturated and trans fats.

Sodium and Salt: Monitor the sodium content of packaged foods, as excessive sodium intake can contribute to high blood pressure and cardiovascular complications. Choose lower-sodium options and limit the consumption of processed and salty foods.

Ingredient List: Review the ingredient list to identify any potential allergens or undesirable additives. Choose foods that have identifiable, whole-food constituents and shorter ingredient lists.

Nutrient Claims: Be cautious of nutrient claims such as "low-fat" or "reduced-sugar," as they may not always indicate a healthier option. Instead, focus on the overall nutritional profile of the food and consider how it fits into your overall dietary goals.

Comparative Analysis: Compare similar products to identify the most suitable option for your dietary needs. Look for products with lower carbohydrate, sugar, and sodium content, and higher fiber and protein content when possible.

Consultation with a Dietitian: When in doubt, consult with a registered dietitian specializing in diabetes management. They can provide personalized guidance and help interpret food labels to support your health goals.

People with diabetes can make educated decisions to enhance blood sugar control and general well-being as they age by reading food labels and nutrition facts. Always prioritize eating complete, nutrient-dense meals, and seek the advice of medical professionals for individualized suggestions.

Tracking Blood Sugar Levels and Meal Effects

Maintaining stable blood sugar levels is crucial for managing diabetes, especially as individuals age beyond 50. Here's a guide to tracking blood sugar levels and understanding how different meals affect them:

Regular Monitoring: Keep a log of your blood sugar levels throughout the day. Test before and after meals, as well as at other designated times recommended by your healthcare provider.

Understanding Glycemic Index (GI): Familiarize yourself with the glycemic index of various foods. Foods with a low GI cause a slower and smaller rise in blood sugar levels compared to high-GI foods.

Meal Composition: Select a diet that is well-balanced and rich in fiber, such as fruits, vegetables, whole grains, lean proteins, and healthy fats. It should also have a lot of complex carbs. This enhances general health and aids in blood sugar regulation.

Portion Control: Be mindful of portion sizes to avoid overeating, which can lead to spikes in blood sugar levels. Use measuring cups, spoons, or visual cues to estimate serving sizes.

Meal Timing: Spread out your meals and snacks evenly throughout the day to prevent large fluctuations in blood sugar levels. Aim for three main meals and 1-2 snacks, if needed, at consistent times each day.

Post-Meal Monitoring: Check your blood sugar levels about 1-2 hours after meals to see how your body responds to different foods. This can help you identify which meals cause significant spikes or dips in blood sugar.

Drink water regularly throughout the day to maintain proper hydration and ensure your body has enough water to function optimally. Stay away from sugar-filled drinks and too much alcohol as these can impact your blood sugar levels and general health.

Physical Activity: Include regular exercise in your regimen; it can help regulate blood sugar levels and enhance insulin sensitivity. A combination of strength training, flexibility training, and cardiovascular exercise should be your goal.

Consultation with Healthcare Provider: Work closely with your healthcare provider or a registered dietitian to develop a personalized meal plan and monitoring schedule tailored to your individual needs and preferences.

People with diabetes can enhance their overall quality of life and more effectively manage their illness by keeping a close eye on their blood sugar levels and knowing how different meals impact them. This is especially true for those over 50.

Dealing with Cravings and Emotional Eating

Managing cravings and emotional eating can be challenging for anyone, especially for those navigating a diabetic diet after the age of 50. ToTake into account the following tactics to assist you in staying on course:

Know Your Triggers: Identify the things that set off your cravings and emotional eating. Is it certain meals, boredom, tension, or sadness? You may create plans to deal with the triggers in an efficient manner by determining what they are.

Make a Plan: Arrange your snacks and meals ahead of time. A balanced diet should include plenty of veggies, fiber-rich carbs, lean meats, and healthy fats. Having wholesome options close at hand can aid in reducing impulsive eating.

Drink plenty of water throughout the day to avoid confusing hunger and thirst. Add flavor with herbs or essences for a calorie-free boost!

Eating with awareness: Engage in mindful eating by choosing your foods carefully, enjoying each bite, and eating slowly. This stops overeating by enabling your body to detect when it is full.

Make Healthy Swaps: Look for more nutritious substitutes for your preferred snacks and sweets. For instance, choose fruit instead of sugary desserts or air-popped popcorn over chips.

Handle Stress: Stress can trigger emotional eating and desires. Look for stress-reduction techniques that are beneficial, such deep breathing, exercise, meditation, or enjoyable hobbies.

Seek Assistance: Never hesitate to ask friends, family, or a medical professional for assistance. Working with a licensed dietician or joining a support group can offer helpful direction and inspiration.

Exercise Self-Compassion: Treat yourself with kindness as you travel. If you make a mistake, move on from it. Rather, concentrate on choosing better decisions going forward.

Get Enough Sleep: Insufficient sleep can cause hunger hormones to become unbalanced, which increases cravings. To enhance your general health and well-being, try to get between seven and nine hours of good sleep every night.

Celebrate Progress: Acknowledge and honor all of your tiny victories along the way. Acknowledge and treat yourself when you make healthy dietary and lifestyle adjustments.

You may follow a diabetic diet after 50 and improve your general health and well-being by adopting these techniques into your daily routine to help you better control cravings and emotional eating.

Celebrating Successes and Progress

As we begin on the journey of managing diabetes after 50, it's crucial to celebrate every milestone and progress made towards a healthier lifestyle. Each day presents an opportunity to make positive choices and embrace the victories, no matter how small they may seem.

From integrating more fruits and vegetables into meals to reducing sugary snacks, every step towards a balanced diabetic diet deserves recognition. Celebrating these successes reinforces the commitment to long-term health and empowers individuals to continue making mindful choices.

Moreover, progress in managing blood sugar levels and improving overall health should be acknowledged and celebrated. Whether it's achieving weight loss goals, lowering A1C levels, or simply feeling more energetic, each improvement signifies a triumph over diabetes and a step towards a brighter, healthier future.

Additionally, celebrating successes can serve as motivation to stay on track during challenging times. By reflecting on past achievements and recognizing the positive impact of healthy choices, individuals can find the strength and determination to overcome obstacles and persevere on their journey towards better health.

Furthermore, celebrating successes in diabetic diet after 50 can be a communal effort, involving support from healthcare professionals, family, and friends. Sharing achievements with loved ones not only fosters a sense of pride and accomplishment but also strengthens the support network essential for maintaining long-term dietary changes.

In summary, celebrating successes and progress in diabetic diet after 50 is essential for fostering motivation, reinforcing commitment, and building a supportive community. Each step towards a healthier lifestyle is a victory worth celebrating, inspiring individuals to continue striving for optimal health and well-being.

CONCLUSION

As we age, the importance of adopting a balanced and nutritious diet becomes increasingly evident. By prioritizing nutrient-dense foods such as vegetables, fruits, whole grains, lean proteins, and healthy fats, individuals can support their overall health and better manage their blood sugar levels. Monitoring carbohydrate intake, controlling portion sizes, and limiting added sugars are key pillars in achieving glycemic control and preventing complications associated with diabetes.

Lean proteins play a crucial role in supporting muscle health, stabilizing blood sugar levels, and promoting satiety. Incorporating sources like poultry, fish, tofu, beans, and lentils into meals ensures a well-rounded and satisfying diet. Additionally, staying hydrated, moderating alcohol consumption, and practicing mindful eating habits contribute to overall health and diabetes management.

However, it's important to recognize that there is no one-size-fits-all approach to managing diabetes. Each individual's nutritional needs, preferences, and health goals are unique, highlighting the importance of a personalized dietary plan. Consulting with healthcare professionals, including registered dietitians or certified diabetes educators, empowers individuals to develop a tailored diet plan that suits their specific needs and lifestyle.

Beyond dietary considerations, maintaining an active lifestyle is paramount for managing diabetes effectively. Regular physical activity improves insulin sensitivity, helps manage weight, and reduces the risk of cardiovascular complications. Incorporating a mix of aerobic exercise, strength training, and flexibility exercises into daily routines supports overall health and well-being.

Managing diabetes after 50 is not without its challenges, but it is certainly achievable with commitment, dedication, and support. By embracing a personalized and sustainable dietary approach, individuals can take charge of their health, reduce the risk of complications, and enjoy a fulfilling and active lifestyle in later adulthood. Empowerment begins with education, support, and the willingness to make positive changes. Let's begin on this journey together, empowering ourselves to live our best lives despite the challenges of diabetes. Remember, it's never too late to take control of your health and embrace a brighter, healthier future.

www.ingramcontent.com/pod-product-compliance
Lightning Source LLC
Chambersburg PA
CBHW051608250726
48653CB00004BA/1405